MILADY STANDARD ESTHETICS: ADVANCED

Student Workbook

To be used with
Milady Standard Esthetics: Advanced

COMPILED BY JUDY CULP

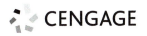 CENGAGE

Australia • Brazil • Mexico • Singapore • United Kingdom • United States

CENGAGE

Milady Standard Esthetics: Advanced Student Workbook
Contributor: Judy Culp

President, Milady: Dawn Gerrain

Director of Content and Business Development:
Sandra Bruce

Associate Acquisitions Editor: Philip Mandl

Product Manager: Maria Moffre-Barnes

Editorial Assistant: Elizabeth A. Edwards

Director of Marketing and Training:
Gerard McAvey

Marketing Manager: Matthew McGuire

Senior Production Director: Wendy A. Troeger

Production Manager: Sherondra Thedford

Senior Content Project Manager:
Angela Sheehan

Senior Art Director: Benjamin Gleeksman

For product information and technology assistance, contact us at
Professional & Career Group Customer Support, 1-800-648-7450

For permission to use material from this text or product,
submit all requests online at **cengage.com/permissions**.
Further permissions questions can be e-mailed to
permissionrequest@cengage.com.

Library of Congress Control Number: 2011941421

ISBN-13: 978-1-111-13911-7
ISBN-10: 1-111-13911-3

Cengage
20 Channel Center Street
Boston, MA 02210
USA

Cengage products are represented in Canada by Nelson Education, Ltd.

To learn more about Cengage platforms and services, register or access your online learning solution, or purchase materials for your course, visit **www.cengage.com**.

Notice to the Reader
Publisher does not warrant or guarantee any of the products described herein or perform any independent analysis in connection with any of the product information contained herein. Publisher does not assume, and expressly disclaims, any obligation to obtain and include information other than that provided to it by the manufacturer. The reader is expressly warned to consider and adopt all safety precautions that might be indicated by the activities described herein and to avoid all potential hazards. By following the instructions contained herein, the reader willingly assumes all risks in connection with such instructions. The publisher makes no representations or warranties of any kind, including but not limited to, the warranties of fitness for particular purpose or merchantability, nor are any such representations implied with respect to the material set forth herein, and the publisher takes no responsibility with respect to such material. The publisher shall not be liable for any special, consequential, or exemplary damages resulting, in whole or part, from the readers' use of, or reliance upon, this material.

Contents

Milady Standard Esthetics: Student Workbook

Contents / v

How to use this Workbook / vii

Part 1: Orientation

1 Changes in Esthetics / 1

Part 2: General Sciences

2 Infection Control / 6

3 Advanced Histology of the Cell and the Skin / 17

4 Hormones / 28

5 Anatomy and Physiology: Muscles and Nerves / 34

6 Anatomy and Physiology: The Cardiovascular and Lymphatic Systems / 40

7 Chemistry and Biochemistry / 46

8 Laser, Light Energy, and Radiofrequency Therapy / 54

Part 3: Skin Sciences

9 Wellness Management / 61

10 Advanced Skin Disorders: Skin in Distress / 66

11 Skin Typing and Aging Analysis / 72

12 Skin Care Products: Chemistry, Ingredients and Selection / 78

13 Botanicals and Aromatherapy / 87

14 Ingredients and Products for Skin Issues / 96

15 Pharmacology for Estheticians / 102

Part 4: Esthetics

16 Advanced Facial Techniques / 112

17 Advanced Skin Care Massage / 124

18 Advanced Facial Devices / 135

19 Advanced Hair Removal / 159

20 Advanced Makeup / 170

Part 5: Spas

21 SPA Treatments / 183

22 Complementary Wellness Therapies / 199

23 Ayurveda Theory and Treatments / 208

Part 6: Medical

24 Working in a Medical Setting / 218

25 Medical Terminology / 221

26 Medical Intervention / 227

27 Plastic Surgery Procedures / 238

28 The Esthetician's Role in Pre- and Post-Medical Treatments / 246

Part 7: Business Skills

29 Financial Business Skills / 254

30 Marketing / 261

How to use this Workbook

This Workbook is designed to accompany Milady Standard Esthetics: Advanced. The exercises in each chapter, which follow the content in the textbook, are meant to test simple recall and reasoning and to reinforce your understanding of the information.

Exercises range from fill-in-the-blank questions, true/false, matching, to more challenging word puzzles, as well as discussion questions that encourage you to apply theoretial knowledge to real-life situations. You may wish to write your answers in pencil, either relying on memory or consulting the textbook. Items may be corrected and rated during class or in discussion sessions with other students, or you may decide to use this workbook for independent study.

We hope that you enjoy using this workbook and that it gives you a comprehensive, study tool for learning about the world of professional skin care.

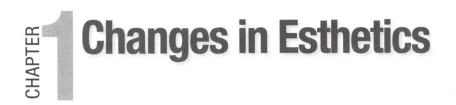

CHAPTER 1 Changes in Esthetics

Date: _____

Rating: _____

INTRODUCTION

Answer the following questions.

1. Why are estheticians in great demand? _____
_____

2. A demand for well-educated estheticians has grown and expanded into the
_____ .

3. What generation has had a huge effect on the skin care industry? _____
_____ Why? _____
_____
_____

THE GLOBAL EVOLUTION OF SPAS AND SPA TREATMENTS

Answer the following questions.

1. How does understanding the history of the spa and spa treatments help the esthetician?
_____
_____

2. Explain two possible origins of the word *spa*:

   a. _____
   _____

   b. _____
   _____

3. Match each of the following words or phrases to its meaning:

   a. _____ *sanitas per aquas*   1. fountain

   b. _____ *spagere*   2. health through water

   c. _____ *espa*   3. to scatter, sprinkle, moisten

4. Name the three water treatments provided in the spa:

a. _____

b. _____

c. _____

5. Before evolving toward the use of baths for relaxation, what was the focus of the Roman bathing culture? _____

6. Name the three types of Roman bath houses: _____

_____

7. What was the purpose of bloodletting? _____

_____

8. During the seventeenth century, the French used _____ springs for drinking cures as well as for _____ and they used _____ springs only for

_____.

9. What did Bavarian monk Father Sebastian Kneipp believe water could be use for?

_____

10. Why did the popularity of spa treatments, such as health and exercise regiments, mud therapy, and balneology, lose ground in the 1900s? _____

_____

11. Worldwide consumers are flocking to spas for _____

_____ , and much more.

ADVANCED EDUCATION AND EMPLOYMENT OPPORTUNITIES

Answer the following questions.

1. Match the following job type with its definition:

_____ esthetician

_____ makeup artist

1. duties may include maintaining records of sales and inventory on hand, demonstrating products, selling to clients, and running the cash register

2. educates clients in the benefits of various cosmetic lines

_____ permanent makeup artist

_____ manufacturer/sales representative

_____ department store cosmetics representative

_____ cosmetic buyer or assistant buyer

_____ manager or salesperson

_____ state licensing inspector or examiner

3. a buyer of cosmetics in a department store, specialty store, or salon

4. specializes in the care of the skin

5. artfully applies cosmetics

6. trained in cosmetic tattooing

7. prepares and conducts examinations, announces and enforces rules and regulations, investigates complaints, and conducts hearings

8. explains, demonstrates, and sells products

2. What are the most common services offered in permanent cosmetics?

_____

3. What can esthetics instructors do to keep up to date on their knowledge?

_____

4. A _____ has the same qualities as a salesperson but assumes more responsibility.

5. If you have talent in writing or journalism, what type of career may you wish to pursue?

_____

DEVELOPING CRITICAL-THINKING SKILLS

Answer the following questions.

1. List the steps for developing critical-thinking, problem-solving, and decision-making skills:

a. _____

b. _____

c. _____

d. _____

e. _____

2. What is a popular method of documenting the critical-thinking process? List and explain the acronym: _____

a. _____

b. _____

c. _____

d. _____

ENHANCING SOFT SKILLS

Answer the following questions.

1. _____ thought revolves around the idea of treating the person as a whole rather than focusing solely on a disease or disorder.

2. List the eight steps to manage negative emotions:

a. _____

b. _____

c. _____

d. _____

e. _____

f. _____

g. _____

h. _____

3. List some of the ways you can release yourself from negativity and distractedness:

a. _____

b. _____

c. _____

d. _____

e. _____

f. _____

PRIVACY LAWS

List the key standards of patient protection:

1. _____

2. _____

3. _____

4. _____

5. _____

6. _____

7. _____

8. _____

2 Infection Control

Date: _____

Rating: _____

RULES AND REGULATIONS GOVERNING WORKPLACE SAFETY

Answer the following questions.

1. Write out what each acronym stands for:

AIDS _____

CDC _____

HAV _____

HBV _____

HCV _____

HDV _____

HIV _____

OPIM _____

PPE _____

2. What is the Bloodborne Pathogens Standard?

_____

_____

_____

_____

3. Give a brief description of each item:

a. Standard Precautions:

_____

_____

_____

_____

_____

b. Engineering Controls and Work Practice Controls:

_____
_____
_____
_____
_____

c. Personal Protective Equipment:

_____
_____
_____

d. Cleanliness of work areas:

_____
_____
_____
_____

e. Hepatitis B vaccine:

_____
_____
_____
_____

f. Follow-up after exposure:

_____
_____
_____

_____

_____

_____

_____

HEPATITIS

Answer the following questions.

1. What does *hepatitis* mean? _____

    Match the various types of hepatitis with the descriptions by putting the number of the description next to the type of hepatitis. There may be more then one response.

    _____   hepatitis A

    _____   hepatitis B

    _____   hepatitis C

    _____   hepatitis D

    _____   hepatitis E

    _____   hepatitis G

    _____   hepatitis I

1. HIV

2. Transmitted via contact with contaminated food

3. A vaccine is available

4. Can be contracted by kissing

5. Caused by poor sanitation

6. Occurs in 25 percent of patients with hepatitis A

7. Occurs in 20 percent of patients with hepatitis C

8. Kills or impairs the immune cells

9. Acquired from blood transfusions and intravenous drug use

10. Can only develop in people who have the hepatitis B virus

MICROBIOLOGY

Unscramble each word using the clues.

1. blmcigooyiro   _____   The science that studies microscopic organisms

2. ornmla frloa   _____   Resident microorganism

3. sdpoamnsueo   _____   A type of resident microorganism

4. trsenntai crmogsminorais   _____   They are easily picked up on hands, clothing, and other inanimate objects.

5. negathpos   _____   Organisms that cause disease

6. yphcclistaooc   _____   A type of resident microorganism

BACTERIA, VIRUSES, FUNGI, AND PARASITES

Label each bacteria and then answer the questions below.

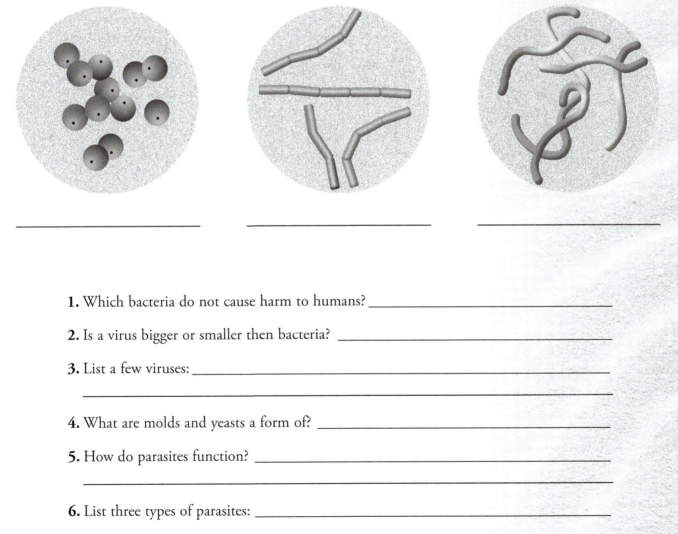

_____   _____   _____

1. Which bacteria do not cause harm to humans? _____

2. Is a virus bigger or smaller then bacteria? _____

3. List a few viruses: _____

_____

4. What are molds and yeasts a form of? _____

5. How do parasites function? _____

_____

6. List three types of parasites: _____

7. When can nosocomial infections appear? _____

_____

Solve the puzzle with terms from the chapter.

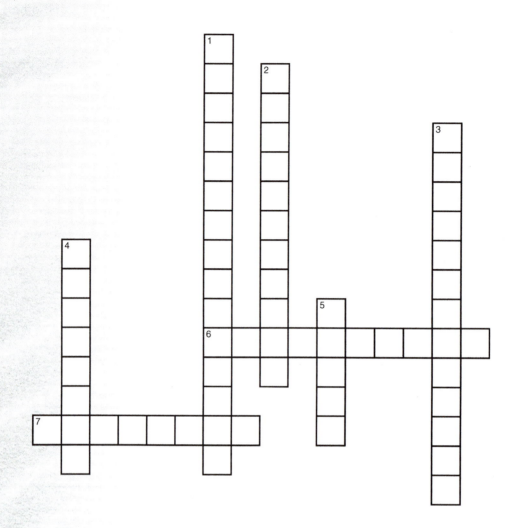

Across

6. A portal of exit.

7. It occurs when the residue of evaporated droplets from an infected person remains in the air long enough to be transmitted.

3. Person-to-person contact.

4. Is another portal of exit.

5. Is a main route for a disease to be transmitted.

Down

1. A microorganism with the ability to spread infection. (2 words)

2. Contact with animal, insect, or parasite.

ASEPTIC TECHNIQUE AS APPLIED TO ESTHETICS

Answer the following questions.

1. What are the two techniques that are used for aseptic control?

   _____

2. What are the five keys of asepsis?

   a. _____

   b. _____

   c. _____

   d. _____

   e. _____

3. What is the definition of *sterile*? _____

4. Sterilized items can include: _____

   _____

5. What are two benefits of hand washing?

   a. _____

   b. _____

6. List 12 times when someone should wash his or her hands:

   a. _____

   b. _____

   c. _____

   d. _____

   e. _____

   f. _____

   g. _____

   h. _____

   i. _____

   j. _____

   k. _____

   l. _____

7. List two ingredients an antiseptic agent should contain:

a. _____

b. _____

8. Put the following list in the proper order:

_____ Use a clean paper towel to turn off the faucet.

_____ Vigorously rub together all surfaces of lathered hands.

_____ Blot hands dry with a disposable paper towel.

_____ Wet your hands with warm running water.

_____ Apply soap.

_____ Thoroughly rinse your hands.

_____ Optional: Apply hand lotion.

GLOVES

Answer the following questions.

1. List the types of gloves that are on the market:

a. _____

b. _____

c. _____

d. _____

e. _____

2. What are some good points for natural rubber latex (NRL)?

a. _____

b. _____

c. _____

d. _____

3. What is a drawback for natural rubber latex? _____

4. What are the benefits of nitrile gloves?

a. _____

b. _____

c. _____

d. _____

5. How can you tell if the material that your gloves are made of is breaking down?

a. _____

b. _____

c. _____

d. _____

e. _____

f. _____

g. _____

CLEANING, DECONTAMIATING, AND STERILZING REUSABLE EQUIPMENT

EQUIPMENT

Put the following list in the proper order for cleaning/decontaming and sterilizing:

_____   Inspect equipment for any residual debris.

_____   Place equipment in a disinfecting tub filled with an EPA-registered disinfectant.

_____   Rinse equipment.

_____   Package equipment with indicators dated for the day of autoclaving.

_____   Place packets ready for sterilization where they will be readily accessible for sterilization process but not where they will become wet.

_____   Thoroughly scrub equipment under water to remove any visible gross debris.

_____   Clean work area.

_____   Rinse equipment again and pat dry.

_____   Ensure that all equipment packages and indicators are properly marked.

_____   Rinse equipment and pat dry.

DECONTAMINATION

Answer the following questions.

1. What is the definition of *decontamination*?

   _____

   _____

2. What are detergents?

   _____

   _____

3. The effectiveness of a disinfectant also depends on other factors, including:

   a. _____

   b. _____

   c. _____

   d. _____

   e. _____

   f. _____

   g. _____

   h. _____

4. Instruments used on clients in a body modification procedure are divided into three categories based on the degree of infection risk when the items were used on clients. Describe each category.

   a. Critical items:

      _____

      _____

      _____

   b. Semi-critical items:

      _____

      _____

   c. Non-critical items:

      _____

5. Describe the levels of disinfection:

   a. High-level disinfection:

   _____

   _____

   b. Intermediate-level disinfection:

   _____

   _____

   c. Low-level disinfection:

   _____

   _____

STEAM STERILIZATION

Answer the following questions.

1. What are the four key things to watch when using an autoclave?

   _____

2. What do indicators respond to? _____

3. What do integrators respond to? _____

4. What should you refer to when using an autoclave?_____

POTENTIAL HAZARDS FOR AN ESTHETICIAN

Answer the following questions.

1. What is an example of a sharp implement that can cause a needlestick? _____

2. What should immediately happen after a needlestick occurs? _____

3. What are the three steps in a screening exposure?

   _____

   _____

   _____

4. What should you look for when inspecting your hands?

   _____

5. The training received at a medical facility may include the following:

   _____

   _____

6. List the basic safety guidelines:

a. _____

b. _____

c. _____

CHAPTER 3 Advanced Histology of the Cell and the Skin

Date: _____

Rating: _____

CELLULAR STRUCTURE AND FUNCTION

Answer the following questions.

1. What does an understanding of the histology and the physiology of the skin provide?

   _____

   _____

2. All cells have the same components, but they differentiate themselves to fulfill different

   _____.

3. Describe selective permeability: _____

   _____

   _____

   _____

4. A cellular membrane is not a single thickness but rather a _____ which is two layers of lipid with water sandwiched in between.

5. _____ make up the lipid bilayer and give the cell its globe-like three-dimensional form.

6. _____ are the communication system between different cells, tissues, and organs and all parts of the body.

7. Where do receptors receive messages from? _____

8. Production of sebum in the sebaceous gland is stimulated by _____ that are received by the receptor sites in the cells of the sebaceous gland.

9. Small structures within the cell that each have their own function are known as

   _____.

10. The structure formed like a maze and located inside the cell cytoplasm is called the

    _____.

11. Very small organelles that help build protein structures from a set of genetic instructions are known as _____ and are the protein "construction department" of the _____.

12. The "lungs" and "digestive system" of the cell are known as _____ and are the energy producers. The mitochondria help to break down simple sugars, fats, and parts of proteins called _____. The mitochondria also take other nutrients, such as proteins, fats, and carbohydrates, and manufacture a substance called _____.

13. The _____ apparatus is a storage mechanism that helps store proteins for later conversion.

14. The "garbage disposal system or recycling center" of the cell, the _____, manufacture enzymes. Describe what these enzymes do. _____

_____

_____

15. Describe the purpose of the vacuoles:

_____

16. Identify each section of the picture below.

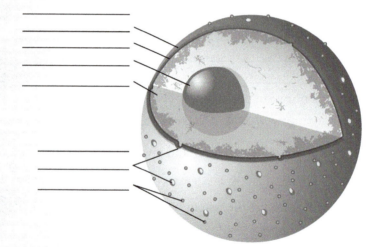

17. The brain of the cell, similar to the central processing unit on your computer, is the _____.

18. _____ within the nucleus are responsible for cellular division.

A BRIEF OVERVIEW OF SKIN STRUCTURE AND FUNCTION

Answer the following questions.

1. What is the largest organ of the body? _____

2. The two major layers of the skin are the _____.

3. Describe the epidermis:

a. _____

b. _____

4. How does the dermis differ from the epidermis? _____

5. List the functions of the skin:

a. _____
_____

b. _____

c. _____

d. _____

e. _____

f. _____

g. _____

MAJOR CELLS IN THE EPIDERMIS

Answer the following questions.

1. What is the major cell in the skin? _____

2. The keratinocyte begins as a _____, also known as a mother cell. It is capable of dividing many times and forming new cells called _____. The daughter cell is transformed into a tiny slab of protein and lipid called _____.

3. Keratin proteins make up part of the _____, which is the support structure in the cell.

4. What are the three main fibers that make up the cytoskeleton?

a. _____

b. _____

c. _____

5. The melanocyte is a cell in the _____ of the epidermis. What does it produce?

_____

6. What is the name of the process that produces melanin? _____

7. Ultraviolet ray exposure causes damage to DNA, which then produces _____ fragments, which triggers release of the MSH.

8. What provides the skin's color? _____

9. What are most skin-lightening agents designed to block and prevent?

_____

10. List the safe agents used for skin lightening:

a. _____

b. _____

c. _____

d. _____

e. _____

f. _____

MAJOR CELLS IN THE DERMIS

Answer the following questions.

1. What is the most abundant protein in the body called? _____ What makes this protein? _____

2. Describe the origin of the fibroblast:_____

_____

3. What are fibroblasts? _____

4. What do mast cells appear to be involved in? _____ Explains what occurs:

_____

_____

5. Leukocyte means _____.

6. Name the two major types of white cells:

a. _____

b. _____

7. How do granulocytes get their name? _____

_____

8. Identify the stain color for each of the following blood cells:

a. neutrophils _____

b. eosinophils _____

c. basophils _____

9. Which type of blood cell is the most abundant type of white blood cell and the most important part of the immune system? _____

10. What is another name for granulocytes? _____

11. The life span of a neutrophil blood cell is _____

_____

12. Which white blood cells are specific for parasitic infections in the body?

_____

13. Eosinophils stay in circulation for _____ hours but can survive for _____ days.

14. What do basophils do? _____

_____

15. List the secretions of basophils:

a. _____

b. _____

c. _____

d. _____

16. _____ provide a barrier between the individual and the environment.

17. The main factor that triggers repair of the stratum corneum is _____.

18. Where are keratinocyte stem cells located? _____

19. Describe the spinous layer: _____

_____

20. What is the major protein formed within keratinocytes? _____

21. The congenital disease known as _____ develops because of defects in keratins 5 and 14 in the _____.

PROTEINS OF THE DERMIS—THE EXTRACELLULAR MATRIX (ECM)

Answer the following questions.

1. The most abundant protein in the body is _____. What is it made by?

_____

2. Elastin is an important protein for:

a. _____

b. _____

c. _____

d. _____

e. _____

f. _____

3. _____ consist of a protein and a complex sugar called a polysaccharide.

4. What is the major function of versican? _____

_____

5. The proteoglycans maintain _____ in the dermis, provide support for other dermal components, and all function as a matrix for _____

_____.

THE CELL CYCLE

Answer the following questions.

1. The final state of growth in cell division is called _____.

2. Identify each of the following bases with its correct abbreviation.

a. adenine _____

b. thymine _____

c. guanine _____

d. cytosine _____

3. A series of enzymes called _____ control much of the process of cell division.

4. How are the epidermis and the dermis regulated? _____

_____

AN INTRODUCTION TO EMBRYOLOGY—THE STEM CELL

Answer the following questions.

1. The study of the very early stages of development after fertilization of any living organism is known as _____.

2. The fertilized egg is called a _____, and it goes through a series of rapid cell divisions at what is called the _____ stage.

3. The three germ layers in the gastrula process are referred to as:

    a. _____

    b. _____

    c. _____

4. The ectoderm germ layer has _____ and produces many tissues and cells.

5. What does the external ectoderm supply? _____

    _____

6. What is the neural crest often called? _____

7. The neural tube provides most of the _____.

8. What comes from the mesoderm stem cell?

    a. _____

    b. _____

    c. _____

    d. _____

    e. _____

    f. _____

    g. _____

9. _____ forms the epithelial lining of the digestive tube.

10. The cells of the ectoderm, mesoderm, and endoderm make up the true _____.

THE MAJOR TISSUES IN THE BODY

1. The body organs are built of _____ *basic tissues. Name them:*

a. _____

b. _____

c. _____

d. _____

2. Match each of the following tissues with its correct description.

a. _____ nervous tissue

b. _____ epithelial tissue

c. _____ muscle tissue

d. _____ connective tissue

1. Separates the underlying organs or tissues from the external environment

2. Provides functions of mechanical reinforcement, transport, and diffusion of nutrients and wastes

3. A highly specialized tissue that is used to transport signals to other organs

4. Provides movement for the body and derives from mesoderm

THE BASIC IMMUNE SYSTEM

Answer the following questions.

1. An elaborate defense mechanism that the body uses to determine self from non-self is the _____ system.

2. Any material that elicits an immune response is called an _____.

3. The body's defense against antigens is _____.

4. What are the two major parts of the immune system?

a. _____

b. _____

5. The active cell in the cell-mediated immunity is the _____. What does the T stand for? _____

6. Cytotoxic or killer T cells do their work by releasing _____, which cause _____.

7. _____ T cells serve as managers, directing the immune response.

8. Suppressor T cells inhibit the production of _____ T cells.

9. What are memory T cells programmed to do? _____
_____.

10. Skin cells contain _____, which are enzymes that destroy bacteria by rupturing their cell walls.

MECHANISM OF EXFOLIATION—THE DESMOSOMES

Answer the following questions.

1. There are at least four types of cellular bonds within the _____.

2. What do tight junctions possibly serve as? _____

3. Tight junctions prevent _____ from entering a cell unless there is _____ for a particular kind of protein.

4. What do adherens junctions provide? _____
_____

5. What do Gap junctions provide? _____
_____

6. The _____ is the major structure that holds the epidermal cells together, and in particular, the cells of the _____.

7. What are the two plates or plaques located in the cell membrane?

a. _____

b. _____

8. The _____ bind the basal layer to the basement membrane through different types of proteins.

9. How much of the stratum corneum is lost each day? _____

10. Enzymes are packaged in the lamellar bodies of the stratum granulosum in an inactive form called _____.

11. When you wish to exfoliate the stratum corneum, what kind of agent must be used?
_____

12. A superficial peel that is about 10 cell layers deep in the stratum corneum will take less than _____ to heal.

SKIN PENETRATION AND PERMEATION

Answer the following questions.

1. Explain what the barrier of the skin controls: _____
_____
_____

2. The pH of the skin is important for barrier _____.

3. Scientists believe that the pH functions to keep the enzymes functioning at the proper level of _____.

4. Proper acid pH is about 5.5, which is the level needed to maintain _____ on the skin.

5. What is a good way to remove skin lipids? _____

SENSORY NERVES AND PERCEPTION IN THE SKIN

Answer the following questions.

1. What is the facial nerve? _____

2. The main sensory nerve in the face is the _____, also known as the _____.

3. Name the three main divisions of the trigeminal nerve:

   a. _____

   b. _____

   c. _____

4. The _____ is the part of the nervous system that is known as the peripheral nervous system.

5. Name the two parts to the reflex arcs:

   a. _____

   b. _____

6. What are the two major functional divisions of the ANS?

   _____

7. The sympathetic division may be considered the _____ part and the parasympathetic division is the _____.

8. _____ are single fibers that join at the hair bulb and wrap around the end of the hair in fine body hair.

9. Describe the function of the Merkel's discs or Merkel cell. _____

_____

10. The _____ is found in frictional areas of the skin, such as the hands, fingers, soles of the feet, and glabrous skin of the toes.

11. The _____ occur in the deep part of the dermis of the palms and fingers near the bones.

12. _____ detect both heat and cold.

13. Where are the end-bulbs of Krause found? _____

_____

14. Nerve endings in the subcutaneous tissue of the human finger are

_____.

4 Hormones

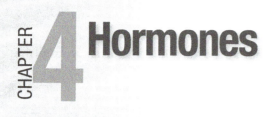

Date: _____

Rating: _____

WHAT ARE HORMONES?

Answer the following questions.

1. List the body functions hormones regulate: _____

2. Which types of glands secrete hormones? _____

THE ENDOCRINE GLANDS

Answer the following questions.

1. How many major endocrine glands are there in the human body? _____

2. Match the following gland with its description:

_____ pituitary gland   a. part of the immune system

_____ hypothalamus gland   b. located just above the kidneys

_____ thyroid gland   c. the ovaries in females and testes in males

_____ parathyroid glands   d. connects the pituitary gland to the brain

_____ adrenal glands   e. best known to produce melatonin

_____ pineal gland   f. secretes trophic hormones

_____ thymus gland   g. regulates growth as well as both cellular
                                              and body metabolism

_____ sex glands   h. are responsible for regulating calcium
                                              and phosphates in the bloodstream

3. Trophic hormones or _____ are chemicals that cause other glands to make other hormones.

4. The pituitary gland produces special hormones that cause:

a. _____

b. _____

c. _____

d. _____

5. The hypothalamus gland controls some involuntary muscles such as the _____.

6. Where is the thyroid gland located? _____

7. _____ are two main hormones secreted by the thyroid gland that regulate the metabolism.

8. How does the calcitonin hormone work? _____
_____
_____

9. Hyperthroidism often results in _____ with the following skin symptoms:

a. _____

b. _____

c. _____

d. _____

e. _____

f. _____

g. _____

10. _____ is an underproduction of thyroid hormones, most often caused by _____, an autoimmune disease that causes an attack of the thyroid so it cannot function properly. Skin symptoms include: _____
_____
_____. Who is mostly likely affected by hypothyroidism?
_____

11. Two hormones needed by the nervous system are _____ and _____.

12. Which gland has a medulla and a cortex? _____

13. _____ could be called the emergency hormone and is secreted when the body is under stress.

14. The main steroid hormones produced by the adrenal cortex are _____ _____ _____. _____ is often called the stress hormone that _____ _____.

15. Where is the pancreas located? _____

16. The specialized cells in the pancreas that produce insulin are called the _____.

17. _____ is a disease that results from the pancreas not secreting enough insulin.

18. Common skin conditions associated with diabetes include: _____ _____.

19. Which gland produces specialized lymphocytes (such as T lymphocytes [T cells] to help the body fight disease? _____

20. The male hormone responsible for development of typical male characteristics, such as a deep voice, broad shoulders, body hair, and other male characteristics, is _____. The female hormone that gives a woman female characteristics such as breasts and helps with the development of the menstrual cycle is _____.

21. _____ is the strongest of hormones and most plentiful until menopause when more *(estrone)* is present; estriol is the _____.

22. _____ is a steroid hormone that helps prepare the uterus for pregnancy and is an important hormone in the menstrual cycle. Progesterone converts to the androgenic estrogens _____.

23. A hormone manufactured by the ovaries is _____, which rises and falls with monthly hormonal cycles and assists in enlarging the pelvic opening during childbirth.

24. The _____, also known as _____, from the pituitary glands causes the production in eggs in females and in males causes testes to produce sperm. The _____ in females causes ovaries to produce progesterone that prepares the uterus for pregnancy, but in males, it causes the testes to manufacture testosterone.

25. _____ hormones cause the actual process of _____ or the release of the egg _____ from the ovary.

THE HORMONAL PHASES OF LIFE

Answer the following questions.

1. During puberty, the production of androgen begins and the _____ produce more sebum.

2. _____ is a sebaceous gland stimulant, and its activity and production causes _____ of the follicles. Describe this dilation: _____
_____
_____

3. In addition, the _____ becomes oilier due to androgen production.

4 Keratosis pilaris is a problem often associated with _____. Describe how it appears:
_____
_____. Describe how to treat it: _____
_____
_____

5. Describe a pregnancy mask: _____
_____

6. What is the cause of a pregnancy mask or melasma? _____
_____
_____

7. Should hyperpigmentation be treated during pregnancy? _____

8. Stretch marks or _____ are marks that occur in pregnant women.

9. What can be used during pregnancy to help reduce the severity of stretch marks during pregnancy? _____

10 An increase in blood flow and blood pressure during pregnancy may lead to the development of _____. Describe this condition: _____
_____

11. Why do varicose veins develop during pregnancy? _____
_____

12. Explain why acne will often flare up after a woman gives birth or while nursing.
_____

13. What normal treatment should not be used to treat acne in pregnant women?
_____

14. Can most routine procedures be performed on pregnant women? _____

PREMENSTRUAL SYNDROME

Answer the following questions.

1. A condition in which some women experience uncomfortable physical changes before menstruation is known as _____.

2. What is the best way to deal with PMS? _____

3. Seven to 10 days before menstruation, women frequently experience _____ .

4. How should premenstrual acne be treated? _____

_____

_____

_____

_____

BIRTH CONTROL PILLS

Answer the following questions.

1. Birth control pills work by manipulating _____ normally associated with the menstrual cycle.

2. Describe the two basic types of birth control pills.

a. _____

_____

b. _____

_____

3. A skin problem often associated with the use of birth control pills is the tendency to have _____ .

4. What type of birth control pills tends to be more aggravating to acne conditions?

_____

5. Another appearance problem related to birth control pills is that of _____ , or melasma.

MENOPAUSE

Answer the following questions.

1. The time in a woman's life when the ovaries stop releasing ova is called _____ .
Describe what happens: _____

2. As menopause occurs, _____ has a strong influence on collagen formation.

3. List what a lack of estrogen may affect:

a. _____

b. _____

c. _____

d. _____

e. _____

f. _____

4. Explain what causes hot flashes: _____

_____

HIRSUTISM

Answer the following questions.

1. Hirsutism refers to _____. Who may experience this? _____

_____

2. How is hirsutism treated?

a. _____

b. _____

c. _____

d. _____

OBESITY, ANOREXIA, AND HORMONES

1. Extremely obese women experiencing a change in hormone levels and activity may also experience _____. _____ women may experience hormonal fluctuations and irregular menstrual cycles.

5 Anatomy and Physiology: Muscles and Nerves

Date: _____

Rating: _____

MUSCLE TYPES

Fill in the missing words.

1. Muscle tissues are referred to as _____. They have the ability to transmit energy, which is called _____, and _____ these enable muscle fibers to react to stimuli.

2. _____ gives muscles the ability to change length, size, and shape and then return to their original form.

3. The two basic types of muscle are _____.

4. _____ muscle fibers are _____, and their movement is _____ and responds _____ to stimulation.

5. Smooth muscle fibers are _____ than striated muscle and react _____ to stimuli; their movement is _____. They have only _____ nucleus per fiber and are _____ in appearance.

6. The cardiac (heart) muscle, sometimes classified as the third muscle, is a special striated muscle found in the _____; its movement is _____.

7. Smooth muscles can be found in internal organs, such as the _____ _____, and are also found in _____.

8. Skeletal muscles are also called _____ muscles and operate _____ due to their thread-like structures responsible for the contractile properties known as _____.

9. Each skeletal muscle is surrounded by a tough outer sheath known as the _____ that connects to _____ and attaches muscle to bone.

10. Muscles are covered, supported, and separated by a fibrous connective membrane called _____.

11. Striated muscle fibers have _____ neurons. In each neuron are synaptic vesicles that store chemicals called _____. Each neuron has an ending, or terminal, that branches out toward the muscle fibers. The region between the neuron

terminals and the muscle fibers is called the _____, also known as the _____.

12. _____ is the neurotransmitter that has the primary function of bridging the synaptic gaps between nerve terminals and receptor sites of the skeletal muscles.

13. The beginning point to a muscle is called the _____.

14. The more movable attachment of the muscle is called the _____.

15. To move a joint in such a way as to increase the angle of the joint is called _____.

16. To move a joint in such a way as to decrease the angle of the joint is called _____.

17. The muscle that goes across the forehead is called the _____.

18. A thick connective tissue attached to the skull that spreads down toward the forehead and connects, approximately, to the frontalis at the hairline is called the _____.

19. The muscle that draws the eyebrows down and together to produce vertical wrinkle between the eyebrows is called the _____.

20. The largest muscles in the body are called the _____ muscles.

FUNCTION OF THE SKELETAL MUSCLES

Match the following muscles to their location or function

A. frontalis

B. aponeurosis

C. orbicularis oculi

D. corrugator

E. quadratus labii superioris

F. orbicularis oris

G. nasolabial folds

H. procerus

I. sternocleidomastoid

J. platysma

K. pectoralis major

L. intercostal muscles

M. internal obliques

1. _____ In the vertex of the skull

2. _____ Located on the anterior of the thigh

3. _____ Muscle in the upper lip

4. _____ Muscle in the chest

5. _____ Forehead muscle

6. _____ Located at the back of leg

7. _____ Around the mouth

8. _____ Muscle of the nose

9. _____ Muscle that rotates the head

10. _____ Muscle originates in the chest

11. _____ Eyelid, upper and lower

12. _____ Makes up the majority of the upper back

13. _____ They run angled to the traverse abdominal muscles

N. trapezius

O. soleus

P. palpebra

Q. quadriceps

14. _____ Draws eyebrows down and in

15. _____ Around the eye

16. _____ Muscles found in between the ribs

17. _____ Marionette lines

Indentify or name the function of the following terms.

1. orbicularis oris _____

2. cardiac muscle _____

3. neuron _____

4. insertion _____

5. frontalis _____

6. frowning muscle _____

7. zygomaticus _____

8. deltoid _____

9. hamstrings _____

10. quadriceps _____

MUSCLES OF THE FACE, NECK, ABDOMEN, ARMS AND SHOULDERS, BACK AND LEGS

1. Label the correct areas with the following muscles: corrugator, procerus, and pyramidalis nasi.

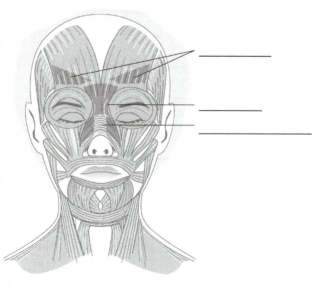

2. Name the two muscles of the neck: _____

3. Name four muscles of the abdomen: _____

_____

4. Name two muscles on the back: _____

5. Name four muscles of the arm and shoulders: _____

_____

6. Name two muscles in the calf area: _____

FACIAL NERVE PATTERNS

Describe what each cranial nerve is responsible for.

1. Cranial nerve VII: _____

2. Cranial nerve V: _____

_____

3. What is Bell's palsy? _____

_____

_____

4. Fill in the missing words in the paragraph using the words from the word bank below:

cranial	motor
brain	head
spinal nerves	12
information	muscle nerves
cranial cavity	

The _____ nerves consist of _____ pairs of nerves that originate in the base of the _____ and emerge from the _____ through various openings in the skull. Some of these nerves bring _____ from senses to the brain and are called _____. Some control muscles (called _____), and others affect glands and internal organs. _____ arise at points along the spinal canal and control sensory and _____ input from the neck down.

5. Fill in the missing words in the paragraph using the words from the word bank below:

upper jaw	motor
maxillary	estheticians
mandibular	ophthalmic
trigeminal nerve	innervate

The cranial nerve V is called the _____. This nerve is important to
_____ and cosmetic nurses because it is intimately associated with the face.
The cranial nerve V has three major branches: the _____ nerve, which
goes to the eye; the _____ nerve, which goes to the _____; and the
_____ nerve, which goes to the lower jaw. All of these branches are sensory
nerves, carrying the perceptions of touch and feeling to the areas they _____.
The trigeminal nerve innervates the cheek and side of the face, the side of the nose and
nasal vestibule, the teeth, and the anterior two-thirds of the tongue. It also innervates
the conjunctiva of the eye, the skin of the lower eyelid, and the tympanic membrane
in the ear. The _____ root of the trigeminal nerve is smaller, extending to innervate
muscles in the lower jaw and floor of the mouth.

Find the key terms from the chapter within the word search using the definitions on the
following page.

```
S Y V G E T R P Z Q N H A M S T R I N G
L I I H A V U H K U A J T H K W W N W V
W M P V W I V I P U B N H L E N J S A S
I D X T U C H V I J O H U L O B C V H F
F S R R F Z A C Z I I W B I C Y D Z E K
H X V L Z S U P T B Y P T A A N K X K H
I F E N T E W C Y N G A U P R G C Y P V
Y D V H F N U P F L X K P O D W Y O F W
E I B Z W D E M A E V B M N I N Y C W A
M E H H D S M X L A M A D E A V H F E P
T K P A W H U F E J L P T U C W C A U W
U M J S Z P W C Z A B A X R T Q S U T N
C B F F T U G Z B A R Y T O F D X K O C
C K N T W I F X F R V Q W S E X M T I X
S F G Q U P P K S N U E K I B V Y H U R
W F L S O A F V J S B Z T S C A P U L A
P J Z B A L A Q W R E W I Z Z K U Z S A
N N K D H Q W D I B B X M Q Q H I I B O
L I H H A E R Q K E N D O M Y S I U M W
X O A J Q N B R A C H I A L I S C J N X
```

1. On the back, or posterior, side of the thigh: _____

2. A movement allowed by certain joints that decreases the angle between two adjoining bones, such as bending the elbow: _____

3. A strong, thick, and flat connective tissue that serves as fascia to bind muscles together or as tendon to attach muscle to bone: _____

4. Flaring cartilaginous expansion on the side of each nare: _____

5. The collar bone and the humerus: _____

6. Muscle cells in the heart: _____

7. Important muscle for arm's ability to flex at the elbow: _____

8. Movement of a limb toward the center of the body: _____

9. Fibrous connective membrane that covers, supports, and separates muscles: _____

6 Anatomy and Physiology: The Cardiovascular and Lymphatic Systems

Date: _____

Rating: _____

THE CARDIOVASCULAR SYSTEM

The following is an overview of the blood, heart, and vein sections. Solve the clues below.
Then look for the answer words in the puzzle.

```
X  G  I  M  C  D  I  A  S  T  O  L  E  B  A  V  Z  Y  Q  Y
E  T  L  Y  X  K  U  N  A  J  R  E  M  R  M  N  Y  N  G  S
F  Y  W  O  S  H  K  F  J  Q  B  P  J  O  D  X  S  X  T  Y
E  L  E  C  T  R  O  L  Y  T  E  S  T  F  B  Z  K  J  X  S
G  O  Y  A  A  O  X  U  S  T  S  H  Q  G  T  G  Y  L  J  T
L  U  J  R  W  A  W  R  O  L  W  H  T  R  A  M  N  B  A  O
I  Z  A  D  H  T  P  A  I  W  B  C  N  A  R  V  Y  U  K  L
C  C  I  I  P  L  M  H  N  K  X  Y  E  N  L  L  X  Q  B  E
P  Q  O  U  E  C  P  P  W  E  E  J  X  U  P  Q  L  Z  P  Z
I  Q  H  M  W  O  V  N  U  H  E  E  M  L  A  Z  X  R  G  R
C  C  T  R  N  T  H  G  M  M  C  W  R  O  J  U  V  M  T  L
H  X  H  I  G  X  B  Q  S  U  M  C  L  C  J  K  O  I  A  F
Q  C  S  N  U  L  G  Q  F  F  X  R  Z  Y  T  F  V  H  B  B
U  O  R  P  K  C  A  U  U  O  Q  H  A  T  F  F  K  V  G  M
E  Z  X  W  A  G  V  A  R  I  C  O  S  E  V  E  I  N  G  L
Z  B  Z  S  E  L  E  K  V  Y  A  E  F  S  C  U  K  Q  X  O
S  P  H  A  G  O  C  Y  T  E  E  V  H  Y  P  O  X  I  A  Q
O  P  C  L  T  V  F  O  X  G  N  C  P  K  N  M  L  A  F  I
N  M  E  M  H  L  F  A  N  T  I  B  O  D  I  E  S  F  P  E
T  Q  B  F  O  I  T  U  L  K  B  L  Q  U  O  D  T  R  F  V
```

1. Phase of relaxation of the heart: _____

2. Proteins that identify and neutralize foreign bodies: _____

3. Anti-parasitic phagocytes: _____

4. Produce antibodies and fight viral infections: _____

5. Deficiency in the blood's ability to transport oxygen:_____

6. Phase of contraction of the heart: _____

7. A double-walled sack that contains the heart:_____

8. Vein that has bulged: _____

9. Cardiac muscle tissue that "pumps" the blood through the body: _____

10. Is found in blood plasma: _____

BLOOD

FACTS ABOUT BLOOD

Fill in the missing word.

1. Blood is considered to have solid, liquid, and _____ properties.

2. Our bodies produce 17 million _____ blood cells per second to replace the ones destroyed.

3. Your body has _____ quarts of blood.

4. The weight of our complete blood supply is roughly _____ of the total body weight.

5. _____ blood is a brighter and more pure red compared with the duller deoxygenated load carried by the veins.

6. Blood temperature is maintained at _____ degrees.

BLOOD COMPOSITION

Circle the best answer.

1. The liquid component of blood is:

    a. erythrocytes   b. albumin

    c. plasma   d. hormones

2. Erythrocytes are also known as:

a. hemoglobin   b. white blood cells

c. red blood cells   d. hormones

3. Leukocytes are also known as:

a. hemoglobin   b. white blood cells

c. red blood cells   d. hormones

4. The cells that multiply at times of acute infection are:

a. basophils   b. hormones

c. eosinophils   d. neutrophils

5. The cells that provide histamine at inflammatory sites are:

a. basophils   b. hormones

c. eosinophils   d. neutrophils

BLOOD DISORDERS

Choose the correct word from the bank of the words to match the definition.

agranulocytes	hemophilia
arterioles	hypoxia
clotting factors	thallassemia
dessication	tricuspid valve
electrolytes	varicose veins

1. _____ Smallest component of the arteries, which connect with capillary beds

2. _____ Condition characterized by incompetent values in the veins, most commonly in the legs

3. _____ Ions required by cells to regulate the electric charge and flow of water molecules across the cell membrane

4. _____ Heart valve that prevents backflow between the right atrium and right ventricle

5. _____ Disorder characterized by deficiencies of clotting factors, reducing the blood's ability to clot

6. _____ Nongranular white blood cells

7. _____ Deficiency in the blood's ability to transport oxygen

8. _____ Specific proteins that act together in clotting; defects in specific protein changes result in clotting conditions such as hemophilia

9. _____ Removal of all fluids

10. _____ Condition characterized by defective hemoglobin cells, resulting in oxygen deficiency

Write a description for each of the following terms.

1. Anemia: _____
   _____

2. Thalassemia: _____
   _____

3. Hemophilia: _____
   _____

4. Leukemia: _____

THE HEART

Answer the following questions.

1. The exterior of the heart is called the _____.

2. The heart is attached to the surrounding organs by the _____.

3. The muscle that makes the heart pump is called the _____.

4. The top two chambers of the heart are called _____.

5. The bottom two chambers of the heart are called _____.

6. Circulation that goes from the heart to the lungs and then back again is called
   _____.

7. Circulation that flows through the entire body is called _____.

HEART DISEASE

Fill in this chart by matching the correct name of a condition to its definition. Choose from the following list.

aortic aneurism
arrhythmia
cardiomyopathy
congenital heart condition
coronary artery disease
heart failure
heart valve disease
pericarditis

	Plaque caused by fat clogs the arteries, restricting oxygen and nutrients needed by the heart; often results in a heart attack
	Inflammation of the pericardium
	Reduction in the pumping ability of the heart, resulting in limited flow
	Heart rate either lower than normal or higher than normal
	Weakened pocket of lining in the aorta
	Gradual enlarging of heart tissues, resulting in heart failure
	A defect in one of the heart's structures, which occurs prior to birth
	Inefficacy of valves in the heart, resulting in backflow or limited flow

THE LYMPHATIC SYSTEM

Answer the following questions.

1. Write a description of the lymphatic system and its primary function. _____

   _____

   _____

2. Label the following on the illustration below: lymph capillaries, lymph duct, and lymph nodes.

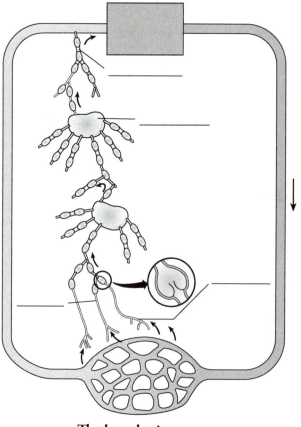

The lymphatic system

3. Blockage of the lymphatic drainage from a limb results in _____, a condition in which interstitial fluids accumulate and the limb gradually becomes _____

_____.

4. The smallest lymphatic vessels are called _____.

5. _____ was the first to employ manual lymphatic drainage.

6. The benefits of lymphatic drainage are:

a. _____

b. _____

c. _____

d. _____

e. _____

f. _____

g. _____

h. _____

CHAPTER 7 Chemistry and Biochemistry

Date: _____

Rating: _____

REFERENCE TOOLS

For each of the following measurements, indicate the appropriate prefix:

One million	*Mega-*
One thousand	*Kilo-*
One tenth	*Deci-*
One hundredth	*Centi-*
One thousandth	*Milli-*
One millionth	*Micro-*
One billionth	*Nano-*

PRINCIPLES OF CHEMISTRY

Answer the following questions.

1. Describe the study of chemistry. _____

_____

2. Describe matter. _____

3. Give examples of elements. _____

4. What is the smallest measurable unit of an element? _____

5. What is the nucleus of an atom made of? _____

6. Do electrons have a positive or negative charge? _____

7.

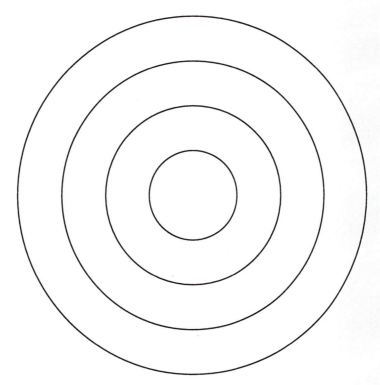

Using the layout, insert the protons, neutrons, and electrons to create a hydrogen atom. Use a red pencil for electrons, blue for protons, and black for neutrons.

8.

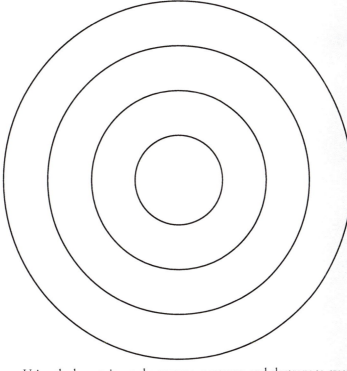

Using the layout, insert the protons, neutrons, and electrons to create a carbon atom. Use a red pencil for electrons, blue for protons, and black for neutrons.

9.

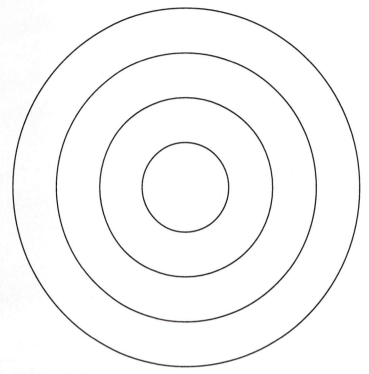

Using the layout, insert the protons, neutrons, and electrons to create an oxygen atom. Use a red pencil for electrons, blue for protons, and black for neutrons.

PERIODIC TABLE OF THE ELEMENTS

Match the element to its symbol.

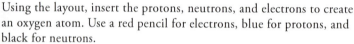

hydrogen _____	Cl
oxygen _____	C
carbon _____	O
sodium _____	H
chlorine _____	Na

Describe each element:

Hydrogen: _____

_____

Oxygen: _____

_____

Carbon: _____

_____

Chlorine: _____

_____

Sodium: _____

_____

CHEMICAL NOTATION

Label the diagram below showing the carbon and hydrogen molecules that we accept as existing there. Use the letter C for the carbon molecules and H for the hydrogen molecules.

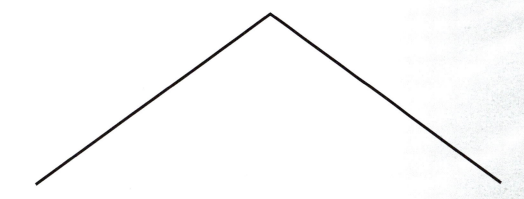

CHEMICALS FOUND IN THE SKIN AND BODY

1. What elements is protein made of? _____

2. What are the building blocks of a protein molecule called? _____

3. What is the bond between amino acid groups called? _____

4. What is peptides linked together to form peptide chains? _____

5. What is a simple unit of a carbohydrate called? _____

PEPTIDE BOND

1. Peptides are made up of _____.

2. How many amino acids are in the human body that make up the 100,000 proteins the body uses? _____

3. Identify the peptide bond by circling and labeling it on this drawing.

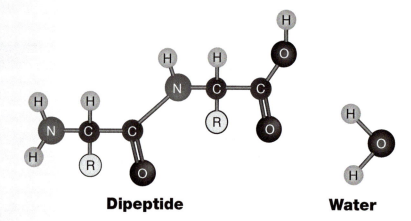

Dipeptide   **Water**

4. Peptide bonds look like this (draw it):

Circle the peptide bond in the following amino acid.

Valine:

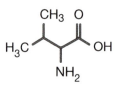

Identify the amino group and the carboxyl group in the following figure.

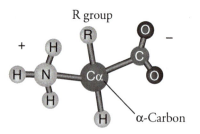

CARBOHYDRATES

1. A carbohydrate is defined as the _____. Units of these sugars are called _____.

2. Two of the most common sugars found in the body are _____.

3. More complex sugars are referred to as _____.

LIPIDS

1. Lipids (fats) are long chains of _____.

2. Most lipids are composed of what? _____ With what at the end?

   _____

3. Fatty acid chains are what type of group? _____

4. Which part is water loving and which water repelling? _____

   _____

5. The goal of lipids in the body is to _____.

CHEMICAL TERMS ESTHETICIANS SHOULD KNOW

Define each term.

1. Proteo: _____

2. Lipo: _____

3. Saccharides: _____

4. Saturated: _____

   _____

5. Aqueous: _____

6. Aerobic: _____

   _____

7. Hydration: _____

8. Homogenous: _____

   _____

9. Suspension: _____

   _____

10. Alcohol: _____

_____

11. Amino: _____

_____

12. Mono: _____

13. Di: _____

14. Carbo: _____

_____

15. Distillation: _____

16. Enzyme: _____

17. Ionization: _____

_____

_____

18. Poly: _____

19. Tri: _____

20. Cyclo: _____

21. Aldehyde: _____

_____

BOTANICAL CHEMISTRY

Fill in the missing word.

1. Metabolites are the substances used by _____ organisms in the process of metabolism.

2. Primary metabolites are required for _____, structure, and reproduction of the plant.

3. Secondary metabolites are the products generated within the plant that are not required for the most basic, _____ sustaining needs.

4. Amino acids are _____ metabolic compounds that are naturally present in the skin.

5. Polysaccharides are made up of a large number of _____ containing monosaccharide units.

6. Alkaloids have _____ effects in the human body.

7. Carotenoids and _____ are found in deep-colored purple and blueberries, green tea, chocolate, and red vegetables.

8. _____ occurs when oxygen reacts at the unsaturated sites, causing a decomposition of the oil and the disagreeable odor associated with it.

9. An _____ is a compound structure that is formed through the reaction of an acid with an alcohol.

ESSENTIAL OIL CHEMISTRY

Use the clues to unscramble each word.

1. pentredio copunmosd _____ Lipids made up of isoprene units

2. enincfraknse _____ Essential oil that has antiviral qualities

3. ngrmea amocilmeh _____ Essential oil that has anti-inflammatory qualities

4. ravledne _____ Essential oil that is a sedative

5. sslegrmaon _____ Essential oil that has antiseptic qualities

6. maotbegr _____ Essential oil that has anti-spasmodic qualities

7. teuplycaus _____ Essential oil that is an expectorant

8. ymeht _____ Essential oil that has anti-parasitic qualities

9. labsi _____ Essential oil that helps a digestive imbalance

10. zeenben grin _____ Responsible for some of the strongest antibacterial and antimicrobial compounds

8 Laser, Light Energy, and Radiofrequency Therapy

Date: _____

Rating: _____

THE HISTORY OF LIGHT AND ENERGY DEVICES

Answer the following questions.

1. What does the acronym *LASER* stand for? _____

   _____

2. On the lines below, write the word that each definition describes.

   a. Small particles of energy _____

   b. The measurement from the distance of the top of one wave to top of the next

   _____

   c. Wavelength distances can be measured in _____

   d. Made up of a multitude of visible and invisible infrared wavelength of light

   _____

   e. All laser light traveling in the same direction _____

   f. Laser light made up of one wavelength and one color _____

   g. When a specific wavelength of light comes in contact with tissue, the photon of light loses its heat energy to the target, or chromophore _____

   h. What vascular lasers seek out _____

   i. Destruction of a target using thermal energy _____

   j. The time necessary for a chromophore, blood vessel, melanin, or hair follicle to lose more than 50 percent of the heat that was produced _____

SAFETY GOVERNMENT AGENCIES

1. Describe the how the FDA determines laser classification:

   _____

   _____

   _____

   _____

2. Describe laser classification by ANSI:

_____

_____

_____

_____

_____

3. Why shouldn't we classify the laser by the associated wavelength?

_____

_____

_____

4. What does LSO stand for? _____

5. List five items the LSO is responsible for:

_____

_____

_____

_____

_____

_____

6. List five items contained in the ANSI Z136.3 document:

_____

_____

_____

SAFETY

Answer the following questions.

1. What is ocular protection? _____

_____

2. How can you control airborne contaminants? _____

_____

3. What type of filter is most recommended for controlling airborne contaminants?

_____

4. How do you prevent the possibility of fire and explosion?

_____

_____

_____

_____

5. In Table 8-1, the Laser, RF, and IPL Safety Policy and Procedure, who does it say should be responsible for selecting the appropriate delivery system?

_____

_____

LASER THERAPY

Answer the following questions.

1. Explain a Photothermal Tissue Reaction:

_____

_____

_____

_____

_____

2. Explain how a vascular laser works:

_____

_____

_____

_____

_____

LASER THERAPY

Fill in the blanks using words from the word bank.

532 nm to 1,064 nm	micro thermal zones
darkening	photomechanical
deeper	pigmented
fractional resurfacing	Q-switched laser
lentigo	water

1. Noting the absorption spectrum of oxyhemoglobin coupled with the depth of epidermal and dermal vessels, lasers ranging from _____ are the most appropriate for vascular lesions.

2. Remember, the longer the wavelength, the _____ the penetration.

3. Photothermal nonablative devices can also be used very successfully for the treatment of _____ lesions.

4. The immediate response of skin experiencing photothermal lasers is either _____, which occurs with melanin break-up, or erythema due to local inflammation.

5. Within 24 hours after the treatment, one can see a crusting or darkening over the _____ or age spot; melanin absorbs the light, which is transformed to heat.

6. Recently, there has been an explosion of new technology in the field of _____.

7. In 2004, Reliant Technologies developed the Fraxel laser, a 1,550-nm wavelength that is absorbed by _____ but can be delivered microscopically in a pixel-type matrix. These columns of thermal energy are called _____.

8. The _____ is the best laser for exploding particles of tattoo ink.

9. The type of laser in question 8 is known as a _____ laser.

10. Draw a line matching the name of the laser to its wavelength.

Q-switched (alexandrite)	800 nm
Diode for endovenous fibers	755 nm
Ruby for hair removal	980 nm
Diode for hair removal	694 nm
Nd:YAG	1,550 nm
Fraxel YAG	1,064 nm

INTENSE PULSED LIGHT

Fill in the blanks from the word bank below.

1995	filter
broad spectrum	hair shaft
chromophore	photodamaged

1. The first IPL emerged in _____.

2. With the variety of skin chromophores, it makes sense to use a broadband light to treat the variety of skin abnormalities seen with _____ skin.

3. Lasers treat one _____ with one monochromatic light while intense pulsed light can target multiple chromophores.

4. The IPL device consists of a flashlamp housed in a treatment head with _____ systems that can select a specific spectrum of visible and invisible wavelengths.

5. A _____ filter spans from 500 nm to 1,400 nm.

6. The _____ will require a longer wavelength such as a red filter.

7. Give definitions for the following terms:

a. Pulsed (1 to 3 pulses):

_____
_____
_____
_____
_____

b. Variable pulse duration:

_____
_____

c. Variable inter-pulse delay:

_____
_____
_____

d. Variable fluence:

_____
_____

e. Large versus small spot size:

_____
_____

f. Skin cooling:

_____
_____
_____
_____
_____

RADIOFREQUENCY DEVICES

Answer the following questions.

1. What is a monopolar RF device used for in surgery centers?

_____

2. What is another name for a dispersing electrode? _____

3. What was the first nonablative monopolar device used for? _____

_____

4. What is used for skin cooling? _____

5. Explain bipolar radiofrequency energy:

_____

_____

_____

LIGHT-EMITTING DIODES (LED DEVICES) AND LOW-LEVEL LIGHT THERAPY

Answer the following questions.

1. What is photomodulation?

_____

_____

2. What is the most common LED color wavelength? _____

3. What else is LED therapy being clinically used for?

a. _____

b. _____

c. _____

d. _____

4. What benefits does a low-level laser light have for a client?

_____

5. What benefits are offered by LED rejuvenation?

a. _____

b. _____

c. _____

d. _____

e. _____

f. _____

g. _____

6. Fill in the crossword puzzle using the clues below.

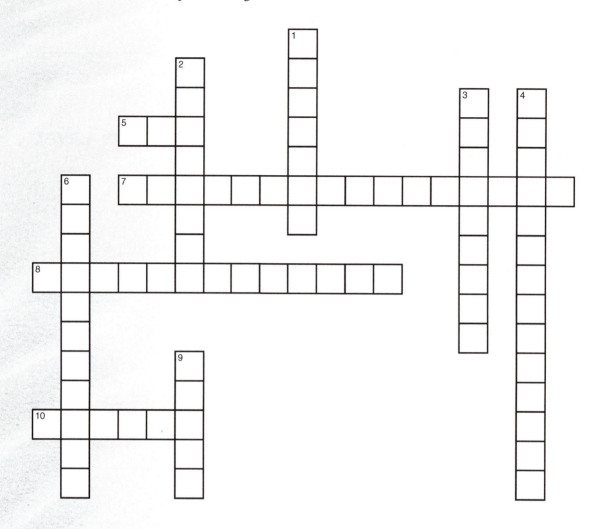

Across

5. Acronym for intense pulsed light

7. Pink, sometimes scaly, abnormal skin lesions that are regarded to be pre-cancerous. (2 words)

8. Parallel rays of light that are traveling spatially and temporally in phase with each other. (2 words)

10. A measurement of a unit of energy from a pulsed laser or light source.

Down

1. Irradiance multiplied by the exposure time, measured in joules.

2. Capable of ablation

3. Metric measurement indicating a billionth of a meter.

4. Protection factor provided by a filter material at a specific wavelength of laser light. (2 words)

6. It is the part of a molecule responsible for its color.

9. Acronym for light amplification of the stimulated emission of radiation.

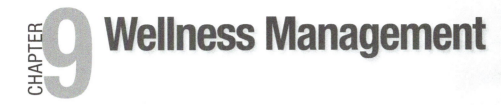

CHAPTER 9 Wellness Management

Date: _____

Rating: _____

NUTRIENTS AND DIET

Answer the following questions.

1. What are the components of food? _____

2. What is a calorie? _____

3. What are the two processes in metabolism? _____

4. The building up of tissue happens during which process? _____

5. The breaking down of tissue happens during which process? _____

THE ESTHETIC BENEFITS OF VITAMINS

Draw a line from the vitamin to its description.

Vitamin A	Helps accelerate hair growth
Vitamin B1	Essential for maintaining natural skin color
Vitamin B2	Also known as riboflavin
Vitamin B3	Helps hair, skin, and nails stay supple
Vitamin B5	Helps control the flow of oil from sebaceous glands
Vitamin B6	Essential in the formation of collagen protein
Vitamin B7	Also known as cobalamin
Vitamin B9	Improves skin ability to take in oxygen
Vitamin B12	Protects against sun damage
Vitamin C	Also known as folic acid
Vitamin D	Slows down skin aging
Vitamin E	Greatly aids in skin respiration

BENEFITS OF MINERALS

From the list provided, fill in the appropriate mineral name with its description.

calcium

Required for muscle contraction, blood vessel expansion and contraction, secretion _____

chromium

An integral part of many proteins and enzymes that maintain good health. Although it is used in oxygen transport, it is also essential for the regulation of cell growth and differentiation.
_____

folate

Needed for more than 300 biochemical reactions in the body.
_____

iron

Is incorporated into proteins to make selenoproteins, which are important antioxidant enzymes that help prevent cellular damage from free radicals. _____

magnesium

Enhances the action of insulin, which is critical to the metabolism and storage of carbohydrate, fat, and protein in the body. _____

selenium

Helps the immune system fight off invading bacteria and viruses and helps wounds heal. _____

zinc

Helps produce and maintain new cells. Also needed to make DNA and RNA. _____

1. How does an antioxidant neutralize a free radical? _____

2. What foods can antioxidants be found in?

_____

3. Why is acne sometimes an indicator of poor nutrition?

_____

_____

4. Which foods can create sluggishness and lead to weight gain?

_____

5. Which foods can deplete B vitamins, resulting in anxiety, fatigue, headaches, and irritability? _____

NUTRITION AND AGING

Answer the following questions.

1. Describe glycation:

_____

_____

_____

_____

_____

2. Which diseases does glycation contribute to?

_____

_____

3. Which foods contain the highest concentration of AGE products?

_____

_____

_____

WHAT WE CAN DO TO SLOW THESE PROCESSES

Answer the following questions.

1. To slow the aging process, cooking temperatures should be kept under _____.

2. Supplements that look promising to help fight AGE are _____

_____.

3. List seven foods that have low concentrations of advanced glycation end products:

_____

_____

SMOKING AND THE SKIN

Answer the following questions.

1. How many years can skin be aged prematurely by smoking? _____

2. Tobacco smoke contains thousands of _____.

3. What affect does smoking have on the capillaries in the face? _____

_____

4. Smokers are at a higher risk for which skin ailments? _____

_____

EFFECTS OF STRESS ON THE BODY

Explain why the following effects happen.

1. Dullness: _____

2. Congestion:

_____

_____

3. Breakouts:

_____

_____

4. Sensitivities and/or irritation:

_____

_____

_____

BECOMING PROACTIVE IN STRESS MANAGEMENT

Explain why it would be beneficial to accomplish the following.

1. Breathing:

_____

_____

_____

2. Put on the brakes:

_____

_____

_____

3. Practice anger control:

_____

_____

4. Go for a walk:

_____

_____

_____

5. Solve the clues below. Then look for the answer words in the following puzzle.

```
C Q L A Z C G O H Q Z A G Z T R B B O N
P D L F P P J O V C F Z L M T W P G Q G
Z I E V O O C N D I X W Y N Y X S E O V
P R X M F L S F G F D R C J I Y C K U D
M N M E G E I V M Q A Q A Z D L Z E P Z
Y N D T N U S C W T G Q T J Y R J W A U
W P W A Q U F C A P E N I V F C B S R H
B H K B J C I A A C A A O J Z O Q O W P
I J I O Q A X L P T I M N J R R W P H U
W K N L A K X R X A A D L R U T M U W Z
I S I I S S L Y C D N B A Q I I Z B N Q
X K A S A D G I G U V M O Z Y S Z T S Q
I A C M Y U H B M E L R R L E O O M Q G
T N I K S Z S Z P Q L F Y Q I L D S T B
V O N V M O S O S A J F L G R S E B R X
I E N T J U N N C N L Z B I Z J M N V E
W S K R Y R Q X E H Q W P R E Z H M U S
V H M Z U S S D O C Q I R A D I C A L W
V U C R A Y A I Y T E R K J N U L H P N
F A I H X O L J Z P P N A F U X L D N F
```

1. Breaks down large units of living matter _____

2. A destructive biological process _____

3. Advanced glycation end products _____

4. A hormone released by the adrenal gland _____

5. Unbalanced oxygen molecule: free _____

6. Process of changing food into forms it can use to provide energy _____

7. Also known as vitamin B3 _____

8. Also known as vitamin B9 _____

CHAPTER 10 Advanced Skin Disorders: Skin in Distress

Date: _____

Rating: _____

THE INFLAMMATION CASCADE

Answer the following questions.

1. What happens when a cell gets irritated? _____
_____

2. The immune system then sends leukocytes, or white blood cells, to the site of irritation, and the leukocytes release another special chemical called a _____.

3. There are different stages of wounds. A compromised epidermis would be a
_____.

4. An example of a Stage 2 wound is a second-degree _____.

5. How quickly does a superficial wound heal? _____

6. What word refers to control of bleeding? _____

7. The final phase of wound healing is characterized by an increase in strength without an increase in collagen content; this is called the _____.

WOUND HEALING

Answer the following questions.

1. What is applied to protect the wound from contaminants, reduce pain, and absorb exudates as the wound heals? _____

2. What should people who smoke be aware of?
_____
_____
_____

3. What effect can the sun have on a wound? _____

SHORT-TERM SUN DAMAGE

Write T next to the true statements and F next to the false statements.

_____ There is no such thing as short-term sun damage.

_____ Reddening of the skin is an example of short-term sun damage.

_____ Sunburned skin will eventually peel due to the extreme dryness.

_____ Sunburn is a non-medical condition.

_____ Treatments for sunburn include cool packs, a cool bath with vinegar added to water, an application of plain yogurt to the area, or the use of over-the-counter anesthetic sprays if the client is not allergic to them.

_____ Many sunburns occur when people are out of their normal environment or are ignorant about sun protection.

_____ You cannot get hyperpigmentation from the sun.

_____ Sun-induced skin discoloration begins in the late teens and early 20s and gets continually worse.

_____ Chloasma (liver spots) are caused by long-term sun exposure.

_____ Tinea versicolor is what many refer to as sun spots or sun fungus.

_____ Tinea versicolor is characterized by brown spots on the skin.

Answer the following questions.

1. How does sun exposure create free radicals?

_____

_____

_____

_____

2. Which cells get chased away by sun exposure? _____

3. What percentage of sun damage do we receive in childhood and adolescence?

_____

4. List some of the effects of the sun on the skin:

_____

_____

5. Define dermatoheliosis: _____

_____

6. What effect does the sun have on the dermis?

_____

SKIN CANCERS AND OTHER SUN-RELATED SKIN GROWTHS

Unscramble the following terms using the definitions as clues.

1. atincic skeartois _____ Rough areas of sun-damaged skin indicated by dysplastic cell growth

2. pldysatcis _____ Abnormal growth

3. ebascuoes ayprheaplis _____ Small, donut-shaped lesions that look like large, open comedones surrounded by a ridge of skin

4. csebrroihe sekiarots _____ Large, flat, crusty-looking, brown, black, yellowish, or gray lesions often found on the faces of older, sun-damaged clients

5. gilenitnes _____ Also known as solar freckles

6. kisn ancerc _____ Condition caused by cells dividing unevenly and rapidly when the genetic material in the DNA has been damaged from the sun

7. thrcyrpyaeo _____ Freezing with liquid nitrogen

8. Describe how a spot of basal cell carcinoma appears:

_____

_____

9. Describe how a spot of squamous cell carcinoma appears:

_____

_____

_____

10. Describe how a spot of melanoma appears:

_____

11. What are the ABCDEs of melanoma?

A: _____

_____

B: _____

C: _____

_____

D: _____

_____

E: _____

_____

ACNE

Use the words from the word bank to answer the following questions.

acne vulgaris	ostium
closed comedones	papule
lamellar granules	Propionibacterium acnes
microcomedones	pustule
nodule	retention hyperkeratosis
non-inflammatory	

1. Acne is a distressed skin condition that results in inflammatory and _____ lesions.

2. The most common form of acne is called _____.

3. The hereditary condition in which cells are retained is called _____.

4. Some researchers believe that retention hyperkeratosis is caused by an inability of the body to produce intercellular structures called _____.

5. _____ are a mixture of dead cell buildup, bacteria, fatty acids from the sebum, and other cellular debris.

6. The opening of the follicle is called the _____.

7. The bacterium that causes acne vulgaris is _____.

8. Small "underground" bumps that are not easily extracted are called _____.

9. A _____ is a red, sore bump without a "whitehead."

10. A _____ is closer to the skin's surface and dilates the follicle opening, relieving the pressure on the nerve endings and resulting in less pain.

11. A _____ is similar to a papule, but it is deeper in the skin and feels very solid and sore.

12. Describe each grade of acne:

   a. Grade 1 acne:

   _____

   _____

   _____

b. Grade 2 acne:

_____

_____

c. Grade 3 acne:

_____

_____

d. Grade 4 acne:

_____

HORMONES

Answer the following questions.

1. Testosterone, an androgen, converts to _____, another form of male hormone, which "switches on" the oil gland.

2. Premenstrual acne flare-ups are caused by the _____ hormone.

3. A sudden flow of sebum in the follicle causes _____.

4. Women who get acne on their chins can be treated with _____ treatments.

5. What are some of the causes of acne breakouts in women? _____
_____

ACNE AND ROSACEA

Answer the following questions.

1. Explain what keratosis pilaris is:

_____

_____

2. Sun exposure may have an immediate drying effect on acne lesions and causes _____, which can add to or increase the chances of acne flare-ups.

3. How does over cleaning the skin affect acne?

_____

_____

4. Describe self-trauma excoriations:

_____

_____

5. Write T next to the true statements and F next to the false statements.

_____ Greasy foods can add to breakouts.

_____ Milk and some milk products have been found to cause acne problems in some women.

_____ Some cosmetics can contribute to acne.

_____ Seborrheic dermatitis is characterized by really oily skin.

_____ Seborrheic dermatitis may be associated with a yeast called pityrosporum ovale.

_____ Perioral dermatitis is dermatitis around the mouth.

_____ Rosacea is characterized by oily skin only.

_____ Clients with rosacea have some flushing and some telangiectases.

_____ Rosacea is a vascular disorder.

_____ The sudden flushing of blood to the face triggers the release of a biochemical within the skin called vascular growth factor.

6. List and describe the following types of rosacea:

a. Erythematotelangiectatic rosacea:

_____

_____

b. Papulopustular rosacea:

_____

c. Phymatous rosacea:

_____

_____

CHAPTER 11

Skin Typing and Aging Analysis

Date: _____

Rating: _____

FITZPATRICK SKIN TYPING

1. Fill in the blank cells in the following chart.

Skin Type	Skin Color	Hair and Eye Color	Reaction to Sun	Common Ethnic Categories
Type I	_____	Blond hair and _____	_____	English, _____
Type II	White	_____ _____	_____ _____	Northern European
Type III	_____	_____ _____ _____ _____	_____ _____ _____	_____
Type IV	Brown	Brown hair and _____	_____ _____ _____ _____	_____ _____ _____
Type V	_____ _____	_____ _____ _____	_____ _____ _____	Asian, Indian, some Africans
Type VI	Black	_____ _____ _____	Tans, never burns, deeply pigmented, never freckles	_____

2. Answer the following questions to determine your Fitzpatrick type.

Points

Question	0	1	2	3	4	Score
What color are your eyes?	Light blue, gray, green	Blue, gray, or green	Blue	Dark brown	Brownish black	

Points

Question	0	1	2	3	4	Score
What is the natural color of your hair?	Sandy red	Blond	Chestnut/ dark blond	Dark brown	black	
What color is your skin (unexposed areas)?	Reddish	Very pale	Pale with beige tint	Light brown	Dark brown	
Do you have freckles on unexposed areas?	Many	Several	Few	Incidental	None	
Genetic Disposition Total						

Points

Question	0	1	2	3	4	Score
What happens when you stay too long in the sun?	Painful, redness, blistering, peeling	Blistering followed by peeling	Burns sometimes followed by peeling	Rare burns	Never had burns	
To what degree do you turn brown?	Hardly or not at all	Light color tan	Reasonable tan	Tan very easily	Turn dark brown quickly	
Do you turn brown with several hours of sun exposure?	Never	Seldom	Sometimes	Often	Always	
How does your face react to the sun?	Very sensitive	Sensitive	Normal	Very resistant	Never had a problem	
Reaction to Sun Exposure Total						

	Points					
Questions	**0**	**1**	**2**	**3**	**4**	**Score**
When did you last expose your body to sun (or artificial sunlamp/ tanning cream)?	More than 3 months ago	2–3 months ago	1–2 months ago	Less than a month ago	Less than 2 weeks ago	
Did you expose the area to be treated to the sun?	Never	Hardly ever	Sometimes	Often	Always	
Tanning Habits Total						

Add all three scores together for a total score: _____ + _____ + _____ = _____

If your score is between 0 and 7, you are a Fitzpatrick I.

If your score is between 8 and 16, you are a Fitzpatrick II.

If your score is between 17 and 25, you are a Fitzpatrick III.

If your score is between 26 and 30, you are a Fitzpatrick IV.

Over 30, you are a Fitzpatrick V or VI.

OTHER SKIN TYPING SYSTEMS

1. The Roberts Skin Type Classification System commonly uses the term i/i/i, which identifies response from _____ .

2. If a female client would be a Fitzpatrick Type III, but her ethnicity is part Cherokee Indian, which classification would you place her in for an IPL? _____

3. To determine post-inflammatory hyperpigmentation, ask _____
_____ If the answer is yes, it is more likely the client will _____ with treatment.

4. Which ethnic backgrounds from the Lancer Ethnicity Scale fall into the rating scale of 4? _____
_____
_____

THE GLOGAU SCALE

Circle the best answer to each question.

1. The Glogau classification system evaluates the level of _____ based on wrinkling.

   a. creasing   b. photodamage

   c. hyperpigmentation   d. pigment

2. Type I on this scale is described as having _____.

   a. wrinkles at rest—you see the wrinkles when the person is not moving

   b. no wrinkles at rest or while moving

   c. wrinkles only in motion

   d. wrinkles as predominant characteristic

3. Type II describes someone who has _____.

   a. no keratosis

   b. acne scarring

   c. early to moderate photoaging

4. Type IV describes someone with _____.

   a. mild photoaging

   b. advanced photoaging

   c. severe photoaging

RUBIN CLASSIFICATIONS

Answer the following questions.

1. Describe Level 1 of the Rubin Classification:

   _____

   _____

2. Which treatments would you perform on a Rubin Level 1? _____

3. Describe Level 2:

   _____

   _____

   _____

4. Which treatments would you perform on a Rubin Level 2?

_____

_____

5. Describe Level 3:

_____

_____

_____

6. Which treatments would be performed on a Rubin Level 3?

_____

ORIENTAL REFLEX ZONES OF THE FACE

Fill in the blanks.

1. In Western schools, they teach that the body is made up not only of solids and fluids but of _____ as well.

2. The vital-energy, as it is called in Western countries, is a very subtle form of energy essential to all life forms. In China it is called _____.

3. The pathways for energy flow within the body are called _____ for acupuncture and _____ for Ayurveda.

4. In traditional Chinese medicine, there are five elements. They are _____
_____.

5. The element that is associated with the energies of the liver and the gallbladder is
_____.

6. The element that is associated with the energies of the heart and the small intestine is
_____.

7. The element that is associated with the energies of the kidneys and bladder is
_____.

8. When one of the five elements is out of balance, undesirable conditions can be created. Name the element that is associated with these various conditions.

Oily skin, blackheads, and hyperpigmentation   _____

Dry, dull, lifeless skin   _____

Lymph circulation problems   _____

Dehydration, lack of tone, wrinkles   _____

Irritated, red, sensitive scalp   _____

ORIENTAL REFLEX ZONES OF THE FACE

Match the zones and organs listed below with the location on the face by drawing a line to the corresponding answer.

between the eyebrows   upper lip

temple areas   spleen

bridge of nose   chin area

lower part of the circle around   liver
the eye

cheeks   gallbladder

hormones   spleen

heart   lungs

ISOTYPES

Answer the following question.

Describe the difference between an estrogen isotype and androgen isotype:

_____

_____

_____

_____

_____

_____

_____

SKIN CATEGORIES

Activity: On a 3" × 5" card, list the priority of skin conditions to incorporate into your skin analysis and used to select what treatment should be performed first:

Skin Condition Priority

1.	_____
2.	_____
3.	_____
4.	_____
5.	_____
6.	_____

CHAPTER 12 Skin Care Products: Chemistry, Ingredients, and Selection

Date: _____

Rating: _____

COSMETIC INGREDIENT CATEGORIES

Answer the following questions.

1. What is the definition of cosmetic chemistry? _____

_____

2. Tell how each term applies to cosmetic chemistry:

   a. Biology: _____

   _____

   b. Chemistry:_____

   _____

   c. Medicine:_____

   _____

   d. Pharmacology:_____

   _____

   _____

   e. Cosmetology: _____

   _____

   _____

3. What are the two basic categories of ingredients?_____

_____

4. Performance ingredients, sometimes referred to as _____, are ingredients that provide the treatment value of a cosmetic formulation.

5. What is a vehicle? _____

_____

6. What is a delivery system? _____
_____
_____

7. What is an emulsifier? _____
_____

8. What is purpose of a surfactant? _____
_____

9. What products are surfactants are most often found in? _____
_____

10. Why are preservatives added to cosmetic formulations? _____
_____
_____
_____

11. What are the color categories? _____

12. Why are fragrances added to cosmetics? _____
_____

13. Describe the difference between pharmaceutical ingredients penetration from cosmetic
performance ingredients: _____
_____
_____
_____
_____
_____

ALPHA HYDROXY ACIDS

1. What is an alpha hydroxy acid? _____
_____

2. Match the acid origin:

_____ glycolic acid   a. _____

_____ lactic acid   b. _____

_____ malic acid   c. _____

_____ tartaric acid   d. _____

_____ citric acid   e. _____

_____ mandelic acid   f. _____

3. What type of client would benefit from mandelic acid? _____

_____

_____

4. Why are glycolic acid and lactic acid popular? _____

_____

_____

5. What are the two main mechanisms of action of AHAs? _____

_____

6. How do AHAs work to promote healthier, softer, smoother, more hydrated skin?

_____

_____

_____

EXFOLIANTS

Answer the following questions.

1. What does an AHA exfoliant accomplish? _____

_____

_____

2. What happens when a client discontinues home-care products for more than three to four weeks? _____

_____

_____

3. What example can you give a client that describes when he or she will see results from an AHA 12 percent lactic acid? _____

_____

_____

AHAs AS MOISTURIZERS

Fill in the blanks.

_____ is an important element in skin moisturization. It is a component of the _____ present in the dermis and epidermis. With _____ and _____, the skin loses its _____ in part because the _____ levels in the skin are significantly diminished, thereby reducing the skin's natural ability to retain moisture. It is now suspected that _____ stimulate _____ of hyaluronic acid and that the "_____" caused by its increase is one mechanism for the decrease in _____ and the _____ effect associated with AHAs.

Clinical studies have also indicated that the _____ of AHAs are independent of _____. Even at concentration ranges of _____ percent, AHA use can greatly increase _____. Studies indicate that _____ the _____ of AHAs in a product appears to follow the law of diminishing returns; when the AHA _____ past a certain point, _____ does not necessarily _____ proportionally. Therefore, _____ AHA products do not necessarily deliver significantly greater moisturization benefit than _____ products. However, _____ do result in more _____, which is one reason for treatment room _____.

FREE ACID, NEUTRALIZATION, AND PARTIAL NEUTRALIZATION

1. What does free acid refer to? _____

2. What is neutralization? _____
_____

3. _____
_____
_____
_____
_____

4. What is the purpose of partially neutralized formulation? _____
_____
_____

ESTERIFICATION AND POLYMERIZATION

1. What is the purpose of esterification and polymerization?
_____
_____

2. What is esterfication? _____
_____

3. What is polymerization? _____
_____
_____

AHA BENEFITS AND USE

Activity: Create a 3" × 5" card for future reference of product concentration with pH levels appropriate for skin type/conditions based on your facility's back bar:

Example of recommendations:

	Acid	Acid Percent	Home Care Product % and pH Value
Aging and Sun Damage	Glycolic Lactic Malic (sensitive)	_____ _____ _____	_____ _____
Dry Skin	Glycolic Lactic	_____ _____ _____	_____
Acne	Glycolic Salicylic Azaleic Mandelic	formulations vary with manufacturer	_____ _____ _____
Hyperpigmentation	AHA Lactic Mandelic	formulations vary with manufacturer	_____

1. List the contraindications of alpha hydroxy acids:

a. _____

b. _____

_____

c. _____

d. _____

e. _____

f. _____

g. _____

h. _____

i. _____

j. _____

k. _____

l. _____

_____

BETA HYDROXY ACIDS

1. What is BHA? _____

_____

_____

2. List commonly used BHAs:

a. _____

_____

b. _____

c. _____

3. What is the maximum concentration of salicylic acid allowed by the FDA for home use?

_____

_____

RETINOIDS AND RETINOID DERIVATIVES

1. What does retinoid refer to? _____

_____

_____

2. What formulation concentration of retinoic acid is usually recommended?

_____

3. What formulation of retinol is usually recommended? _____

4. Why are retinoids the most effective ingredient for improving the signs of skin aging?

_____

_____

_____

_____

5. Why are retinoids effective for acne treatments? _____

_____

_____

_____

_____

_____

FREE RADICALS

Answer the following questions.

1. What is a free radical? _____

_____

_____

_____

_____

_____

_____

2. Free radicals attack proteins and damage the framework and functioning of the skin. List the body components that free radicals negatively affect:

a. _____

b. _____

c. _____

d. _____

e. _____

SUNSCREENS

1. List the sunscreen organic chemicals: _____

_____

2. List the sunscreen inorganic chemicals (mineral ingredients): _____

_____

3. As of when is the U.S. FDA Final Rule on Sunscreen Labeling effective?

_____

4. What does term "broad spectrum SPF" refer to? _____

_____

_____

_____

_____

ANTIOXIDANTS

Unscramble the following antioxidants.

nviamit C   _____

itvmnai E   _____

teab eenracot   _____

xidupsreoe mustaidse   _____

rppoec   _____

degaperse traextc   _____

cyprinanothoadnsi   _____

heppoylnosl   _____

hroltocpeo   _____

Lsocracbi diac   _____

lgcilae acdi   _____

phaal copiil daci   _____

MOISTURIZERS—THE ESSENTIAL NEED FOR SKIN HYDRATION

List the functions of the following ingredients and give examples of each.

1. Emollients: _____

_____

2. Humectants: _____

_____

3. Occlusive lipids: _____

_____

4. High-molecular-weight ingredients: _____

_____

_____

UNDERSTANDING ORGANIC

1. Define *organic*: _____

_____

_____

_____

2. What does *organically grown* mean? _____

_____

3. Describe natural ingredients: _____

_____

4. For what type of products does the government issues certificates? _____

_____

NANOTECHNOLOGY

1. What is nanotechnology? _____

_____

2. What is a nano element? _____

_____

_____

3. Describe nanomaterials and their importance in cosmetics applications:

_____

_____

_____

4. List examples of how nanotechnology is being used in products: _____

_____

_____

13 Botanicals and Aromatherapy

Date: _____

Rating: _____

WHAT ARE BOTANICAL INGREDIENTS?

Answer the following questions.

1. What role do botanical fixed oils, essential oils, herbal extracts, and other plant-based therapies have on cosmetic preparations?

_____

2. What does *botanical* mean? _____

3. The benefits of plant extracts include:

a. _____

b. _____

c. _____

d. _____

e. _____

f. _____

g. _____

h. _____

i. _____

j. _____

k. _____

4. In what skin care applications are plant derivatives used?

a. _____

b. _____

c. _____

d. _____

e. _____

f. _____

g. _____

5. Define *whole extract*: _____
_____

6. Define and give an example of an isolate: _____
_____
_____

7. What is a tincture? _____
_____

8. How do you make an herbal infusion? _____
_____

9. What is a fixed oil? _____

10. Give examples of fixed oils: _____

11. How do they get the oils out of the above natural substances? _____

12. What is a method of extraction that is popular in the fragrance industry?
_____

BOTANICALS FOR SKIN CARE

Fill in the missing cells in the chart.

Name of Botanical	Properties	Uses
Aloe Vera	Anti-inflammatory, regenerative, moisturizing, soothing, healing	Burns, _____ _____
Arnica Montana	Anti-inflammatory	_____ _____
Bamboo	_____ _____	_____ _____
Cocoa (butter and powder)	Anti-inflammatory, antioxidant, emollient, regenerative	General skin care and conditioning, _____ _____

Name of Botanical	Properties	Uses
Comfrey	_____ _____	_____ _____
Cranberry seed oil	_____ _____ _____	_____ _____ _____
Green tea	Anti-inflammatory, _____ _____ , circulatory stimulant	_____ _____ _____
Kelp	Wound healing, detoxifying	_____ _____ _____
Marigold	_____ _____ _____	_____ _____ _____
Shea butter	_____ _____ _____	_____ _____ _____

AROMATHERAPY AND ESSENTIAL OILS

Answer the following questions.

1. How does a practitioner use essential oils effectively?

_____

_____

_____

2. When did the practice of aromatherapy begin?

_____

_____

_____

_____

_____

3. What are essential oils?

_____

_____

4. What is the olfactory system? _____

5. What is homeostasis?

_____

_____

6. What does the limbic system do?

_____

7. What role does the hypothalamus play?

_____

_____

8. What topical applications can be achieved with essential oils?

a. _____

b. _____

c. _____

d. _____

e. _____

f. _____

ESSENTIAL OIL CHEMISTRY

Fill in the missing cells in the chart.

Chemical Family	Essential Oils with Influential Amounts	Properties	Cautions	Examples of Individual Components within the Family
Monoterpene hydrocarbons (the most abundant compounds in essential oils)	Needle tree oils, such as cypress, pine, and spruce Citrus oils such as grapefruit, lemon, and orange Frankincense	Diuretic, antiviral, stimulant, tonic	_____ _____ _____ _____ _____ _____ _____	Alpha-pinene limonene

Chemical Family	Essential Oils with Influential Amounts	Properties	Cautions	Examples of Individual Components within the Family
Sesquiterpene hydrocarbons	German chamomile, _____ _____	Anti-allergic, anti-inflammatory, cooling		Chamazulene beta-caryophyllene
Monoterpene alcohols _____ _____ _____ _____	Lavender, MQV _____ _____ _____ palmarosa, _____ _____	_____ _____ _____ _____ _____ _____ _____		Linalool borneol menthol terpinen-4-ol
Sesquiterpene alcohols	_____ _____ _____	_____ _____ _____ _____ _____ _____ _____		Cedrol santalol-alpha-bisabolol
Aldehydes	_____ _____ _____ _____	_____ _____ _____ _____	_____ _____ _____ _____	Citral, citronallal
Esters	_____ _____ _____ _____ _____ _____	_____ _____ _____ _____		Geranyl acetate linalyl acetate methyl acetate

Chemical Family	Essential Oils with Influential Amounts	Properties	Cautions	Examples of Individual Components within the Family
Ketones	_____ _____ _____ _____ _____	_____ _____ _____	_____ _____ _____ _____ _____ _____ _____ _____ _____ _____ _____ _____ _____ _____ _____ _____ _____ _____	itallidone thujone verbenone
Lactones	_____ _____	_____	Used with caution	alpha-lactone
Oxide	_____ _____ _____	_____ _____		1, 8 cineole rose oxide
Phenols	_____ _____	_____ _____ _____ _____ _____	Skin irritant	carvacrol thymol
Phenylpropanes	_____ _____	_____ _____	Skin irritant. Liver toxin at high dosages	cinnamic aldehyde euganol

Chemical Family	Essential Oils with Influential Amounts	Properties	Cautions	Examples of Individual Components within the Family
Ether (phenolpropane derivatives)	_____ _____ _____	_____ _____ _____ _____	Toxic to the nervous system at very high dosages	anethol methyl chavicol myristicin

1. List the healing properties for each essential oil:

Cedarwood: _____

Cape chamomile: _____

Eucalyptus: _____

Geranium: _____

Grapefruit: _____

Helichrysum: _____

Lavender: _____

Neroli: _____
_____

Niaouli: _____

Palmarosa: _____
_____

Rosemary verbenone type: _____

Australian sandalwood: _____
_____

Ylang ylang: _____

BLENDING ESSENTIAL OILS

List the uses of essential oils:

1. _____

2. _____

3. _____

4. _____

5. _____

6. _____

7. _____

8. _____

9. _____

10. _____

11. _____

CARRIER OILS

1. List the skin benefits for each carrier oil:

a. Coconut oil: _____

b. Jojoba oil: _____

c. Kukui nut: _____

d. Olive oil: _____

e. Raspberry seed oil: _____

f. Rose hip seed oil: _____

g. Sunflower seed oil: _____

2. Search for the following terms in the word search puzzle below.

absolutes	isolate
allantoin	jojoba oil
emulsifier	phytotherapy
essential oil	refined
fixed oil	synergy

```
X T E W C O D K E Q V C G D S O E O I X
Z H S B W C W G B W Z X H Z S F A F O I
E A C Y P M E B E T R E R W Q Y I Z J D
D P Y G E E B U K K S F M Z K O N P B S
O D G Z D H M I A C C P U Q A D Z P W E
K R R G E L A Y B Q E U U Q U J H M G T
F J D G F F S H R E I F I S L U M E T U
O F M F D Z O K C E N B V J G Y F P W L
V C G U R E F I N E D T L U O K H G C O
P I I K A V R A N J Y Y G U B Y T G M S
C E S S E N T I A L O I L F T W P W B B
H B P T X U G R N V R I Y O Q K I H S A
Q L R V U T Y I X W W E T Q B K J E Y E
H T M L T H X J C C T H G I S B Q A G C
P S H X K I E Z C M E Z N Z R U U X R I
N I O T N A L L A R F I X E D O I L E K
P T H T C Q L M A P W L D Z S P G V N M
F G A N D U S P Q N G X B I Q K R K Y I
Z I C N C B Y H N I S O L A T E Z Q S M
U W P D J O J O B A O I L X T V U E V Z
```

14 Ingredients and Products for Skin Issues

Date: _____

Rating: _____

CLEANSERS

Fill in the blanks in each sentence.

1. Regardless of its texture, a cleanser should not be drying but rather help preserve the skin's natural protective barrier _____ .

2. In places where the water is very _____, sometimes called "_____" water, it is best to rinse cleansers with _____ can be drying or increase the feeling of dryness for those with dry skin.

3. Cleansers with _____ have a multi-purpose characteristic as they cleanse, _____, and, in most cases, also _____.

TONERS

Answer the following questions.

1. Name three reasons to use toners:

a. _____

b. _____

_____

c. _____

_____

CREAMS

Fill in the blanks in each sentence.

1. What performance ingredients are used in eye creams? _____

2. Creams with nourishing or _____, such as those with retinol or other retinoids, tend to be used at _____ .

3. For a descriptive purpose, we can divide creams into _____ and _____, which would include the "_____" category, plus neck, eye and body creams.

PERFORMANCE CREAMS: DAY AND NIGHT

Fill in the blanks in each sentence.

1. Performance creams usually contain "_____" ingredients oriented to a specific skin type and condition. They may contain _____ _____ and/or retinoids _____ for anti-aging.

2. Acne treatment could include the same set of ingredients (though in different proportions), plus _____ and other problem-solving ingredients.

3. For _____ creams could also include _____ and a range of botanicals such as _____.

TRADITIONAL CREAMS: DAY AND NIGHT

Fill in the blanks in each sentence.

1. Traditional day creams tend to be _____, without high concentrations of "_____" ingredients.

2. Traditional night creams, also referred to as "_____," are generally designed to help _____ at night, a time when normal _____ is taking place all over the body, including the skin.

3. Night creams are often _____ in consistency and texture than their daytime counterparts. They normally contain more _____ than day creams.

4. Nourishing creams will contain _____ and may contain _____ together with other botanical ingredients including _____ and _____.

MOISTURIZERS

Fill in the blanks in each sentence.

1. Moisturizers, also called _____, are an extremely important product category because they can provide a great deal of _____ activity for young and mature clients alike.

2. A moisturizer should include a number of appropriate, moisturizing performance components. In addition, moisturizers are an ideal medium for incorporating a wide range of antioxidants including botanical antioxidants like _____ _____ as well as other appropriate _____. _____ are being added to a wide range of products, and their incorporation into moisturizers can be an invaluable _____ tool.

ABOUT AMPOULES AND SERUMS

Fill in the blanks in each sentence.

1. Ampoules are generally sealed glass vials of _____, designed to give ultra-intensive treatment to the skin. They often contain _____ of _____ ingredients in a _____, though occasionally they are in an oil base.

2. Serums contain _____ ingredients, often in _____ or other advanced delivery systems. They tend to contain specialty ingredients including _____ extracts. Like ampoules, they are applied under a cream or lotion.

MASKS AND EXFOLIANTS

Fill in the blanks in each sentence.

1. Masks are designed to treat a variety of skin problems, from _____ _____. They are formulated with less water than creams, lotions, and fluids and are considerably _____ than any of these products.

2. Oily skin: Masks may contain _____. These clays are helpful in absorbing _____.

3. Acne-prone skin: A mask might contain _____ plus _____ for _____ action.

4. _____ masks often contain large amounts of _____.

5. _____ can be mechanical or chemical. _____ exfoliants usually come in the form of _____. They are usually water-based products with a _____ mixed with some sort of abrasive agent such as _____ granules, or _____ beads.

6. _____ exfoliants are a _____ exfoliant usually based on botanicals and are milder than mechanical exfoliants. They are _____ and work by loosening _____ so that they can be rinsed away

7. Other _____ exfoliators are usually based on _____ _____. In the case of alpha hydroxy acids, they exfoliate the excess accumulation of _____.

SUNLESS TANNERS

Fill in the blanks in each sentence.

1. There are three primary categories of such products: _____
_____.

2. _____ is a term that includes all forms of tanning beds and sunlamps. They do not
prevent the _____ associated with _____, nor do they prevent the
production of _____.

3. _____ are products that give the skin a tanned appearance without having
been exposed to the _____ or other sources of _____. _____
_____ is the most commonly used ingredient in sunless tanners.

4. Bronzers provide a _____ tanned look and tend to be _____,
_____, and other such cosmetics that can be washed off. Some contain
_____, providing a longer-lasting "tanned" appearance.

LINE SELECTION FOR DESIGNING A SUCCESSFUL HOME-CARE REGIMEN

Activity: Using the products in your facility, design a 3" × 5" card with specific skin
conditions and product recommendations:

	Dry/Mature	Sensitive	Normal/Combo	Oily/Acne	Hyper-pigmentation
Cleanser					
Enzyme					
Mask					
Serum					
Moisturizer					

Fill in the missing performance ingredient names and ingredient functions or actions:

Ingredient Name	Ingredient Function/Action
Agua (water)	A major component in product formulations.
_____	Humectant. It is water binding and promotes _____.
Butylene glycol	Solvent. _____ action.
_____	Skin conditioning.
Ascorbic acid	_____

Ingredient Name	Ingredient Function/Action
_____	Natural emollient. Acts as a moisturizer.
Glyceryl stearate	_____
PEG 100 stearate	Stabilizer. Emulsifying agent.
Sorbitan stearate	Emulsifier for _____ and lotions.
Tocopherol acetate	_____
_____	Antioxidant.
Ubiquinone	Antioxidant.
Steareth 2	Emulsifier.
Acrylates C10-30	Emulsifier.
Acrylates crosspolymer	Reduces skin shine through oil absorption. Gives a pleasant feel to the product. Improves the functioning of other ingredients. Can form a protective barrier against moisture loss.
Triethanolamine	Emulsifier. pH adjuster.
Disodium EDTA	_____
Xanthan gum	Texturizing and gelling agent.
_____	Preservative.
_____	Preservative.
Imidazolinidinyl urea	Antibacterial preservative.

• Remember that the _____ of a specific ingredient present in a product is represented by its _____ in the product label. The _____ ingredient is the one representing the _____ in the formulation; usually this is _____. Ingredients must be listed in _____ of predominance. In the case of a _____—an extract or other ingredient carried in water—it may be listed near the _____ because of its water content, although the actual extract is in the formula at a much _____.

HOW PRODUCTS ARE DEVELOPED

1. Name the steps for developing a product:

a. _____

b. _____

c. _____

d. _____

e. _____

f. _____

g. _____

CHAPTER 15 Pharmacology for Estheticians

Date: _____

Rating: _____

THE FDA AND DRUGS

Answer the following questions.

1. What does FDA stand for? _____

2. When and why did the FDA come into being? _____
_____
_____
_____

3. What is the definition of a prescription? _____
_____
_____
_____
_____

DRUG CLASSIFCATION

Fill in the information that is missing from the chart.

Classification	Purpose
Analgesics (narcotic and non-narcotic)	Drugs to relieve pain
Antacids	_____
Antianxiety drugs	_____
Antiarrhythmics	_____
Antibiotics	_____ _____
Anticoagulants	_____
Anticonvulsants	_____
Antidepressants	_____

Classification	Purpose
Antidiarrheals	
Antiemetics	
Antifungals	Treat fungal infection
Antihistamines	
Antihypertensives	
Anti-inflammatories	Reduce tissue swelling, reduce pain
Antipsychotics	
Antipyretics	Reduce fever
Beta blockers	
Bronchodilators	
Corticosteroids	
Cough suppressants	
Cytotoxics	Kill cancer cells
Decongestants	
Diuretics	
Expectorants	
Hormones	
Hypoglycemics	
Immunosuppressives	
Laxatives	
Muscle relaxants	
Sedatives, hpnotics	
Thrombolytics	
Vitamins	

COMMON ORAL PRESCRIPTION DRUGS THAT MAY AFFECT THE SKIN

Fill in the information that is missing from the chart.

Classification	Medication Examples
Antidepressants	Prozac, Zoloft
Antibiotics	_____
Antivirals	Zovirax, Valtrex
Antifungals	_____
Diuretics	_____
Antihypoglycemic	_____
_____	Estrogen, progesterone
Oral contraceptives	Many varieties

COMMON TOPICAL DRUGS PRESCRIBED FOR SKIN DISORDERS

Fill in the information that is missing from the chart.

Classification	Examples of Reasons for Prescribing	Medication Examples	Skin Side Effects
Anti-aging drugs	Reduces fine wrinkles and hyperpigmentation	_____	_____ _____ _____ _____ _____ _____ _____ _____ _____
Anti-acne drugs	_____ _____ _____ _____	_____	Same as Renova
Antibiotics	_____	Cleocin T	Dry, scaly skin

Classification	Examples of Reasons for Prescribing	Medication Examples	Skin Side Effects
Antifungals	Treatment of *Tinea* infections and cutaneous candidiasis	Lamisil, Lotrimin, Loprox	_____ _____ _____ _____ _____
Anesthetics	Relief of pain related to arthritis and muscular aches	_____	_____ _____ _____
Corticosteroids	_____ _____ _____ _____	Aclovate	Skin atrophy, contact dermatitis, stretch marks, enlarged blood vessels, hair loss, pigment changes, secondary infections

COMMON OVER-THE-COUNTER DRUGS THAT MAY AFFECT THE SKIN

Fill in the information that is missing from the chart.

Classification	Common Use	Common Products	Skin Side Effects
Analgesics	_____	Ibuprofen (Motrin)	_____
Antacids	Relieve indigestion/heartburn	Tums, Mylanta	None known
H2 antagonists (histamine blockers)	Treat gastro-esophageal reflux, ulcers	_____	_____
Proton pump inhibitors	Treat various gastric disorders	_____	_____
Antidiarrheals	Treat minor diarrhea	_____	_____

HORMONE AND CONTRACEPTIVES

Fill in the information that is missing from the chart.

Classification	Prescription Hormone Examples	Skin Side Effects
_____	Calcitonin (Calcitonin sasal sprays), danazol (Danacrine), desmopressin (DDAVP oral or nasal spray), estradiol valerate, estradiol/ethinyl estradiol, estropipate, Premarin, fludrocortisone, insulin, leuprolide (injected), levothyroxine (Levoxyl, Synthroid), liothyronine (Cytomel), liotrix (Thyrolar), megestrol (Megace), nafarelin nasal (Synarel), progesterone, vasopressin	Acne, flushing of the face, hirsutism, oily skin, pruritus, photosensitivity, rash (rare) Transdermal estradiol: skin irritation, redness Estradiol and progesterone: dark patches on exposed skin (melasma) Fludrocortisone: changes in skin appearance (e.g., fatty areas, color changes, thinning), easy bleeding/ bruising, slow wound healing, skin and nasal sores, puffy face (refer client to physician) Vasopressin: pale skin, pale skin around mouth, sweating
Oral contraceptives	All containing any form of estradiol or estradiol/ethinyl estradiol Common brand names: Estrostep, Ortho Tri-Cyclen, Ortho-Novum, Tri-Norinyl, Nor-OD, Yaz	_____

MEDICATIONS THAT AFFECT THE BLOOD

Fill in the information that is missing from the chart.

Classification	Medication Example	Skin Side Effects
Antihyperlipidemics (lipid-lowering agents)	_____	_____
Anticoagulants	Coumadin (warfarin)	_____ _____
_____	Aspirin, Plavix, Ticlid, Effient	_____ _____ _____ _____ _____

COMMON DRUGS USED TO TREAT HEART CONDITIONS

1. Draw a line to match the terms to their definitions.

hypertension   By injection

acute coronary syndrome   Placed under the tongue

angina   High blood pressure

antianginals   Medical term for chest pain

sublingual   Problems associated with blood flow to the heart

parenteral   Drugs used to treat angina

2. Fill in the information that is missing from the chart.

Drug Category	Example	Common Skin Effects
Beta blockers	_____ _____	_____ _____ _____
Calcium channel blockers	_____, isradipine, nicardipine, verapamil	_____
Nitrates	isosorbide mononitrate, isosorbide dinitrate, _____	_____ _____ _____
Antiarrhythmics	disopyramide, moricizine, procainamide, quinidine, fosphenytoin, mexiletine, tocainide, acebutolol, diltiazem, atropine	_____ _____ _____ _____
Antihypertensives	clonidine, eplerenone, benazepril, captopril, lisinopril, moexipril, ramipril, guanfacine, methyldopa, _____	_____ _____

MEDICATIONS FOR RESPIRATORY DISORDERS

Draw a line to match the terms to their definitions.

antihistamines   A respiratory condition

antiasthmatics   Chemical mediator

bronchodilators   An example is levalbuterol

asthma   To prevent asthmatic conditions

antigen   Used to block histamine reactions

histamine   Invading substance

MEDICATIONS USED TO TREAT GASTROINTESTINAL AND URINARY TRACT DISORDERS

Fill in the information that is missing from the chart.

Classification	Medication Example	Skin Side Effects
Anticholinergics	Hyoscyamine _____, tolteradine _____	_____
Antidiarrheals	Diphenoxylate with atropine _____, loperamide _____	_____ _____
Antiemetics	Ondansetron (Zofran), promethazine (Phenergan)	Rare hypersensitivity reaction: (rash, pruritus, flushing, sweating, photosensitivity, urticaria)
_____	Lansoprazole (Prevacid), nizatidine (Axid), omeprazole (Prilosec), rabeprazole (Aciphex)	_____ _____

MEDICATIONS USED TO TREAT MENTAL ILLNESS

Answer the following questions.

1. List five anxiety disorders:

a. _____

b. _____

c. _____

d. _____

e. _____

2. What type of medication would someone with anxiety disorder take? _____

3. List antidepressants used today:

a. _____

b. _____

c. _____

d. _____

4. List the skin disorders that match the following group of medications:

Medications Used to Treat Mental Illness, Epilepsy, and Sleep Disorders

Classification	Medication Examples	Skin Side Effects
Antianxiety drugs	Chlordiazepoxide (Librium)	Rash
Anticonvulsants	Carbamazepine (Tegretol), phenobarbital, phenytoin (Dilantin), divalproex sodium (Depakote)	_____ _____ _____
_____	Citalopram _____, paroxetine _____, sertraline _____, mirtazapine _____, bupropion _____	_____ _____ _____
Antipsychotics	Aripiprazole (Abilify), clozapine (Clozaril), fluphenazine (Prolixin), resperidone, (Risperdal), ziprasidone (Geodon), quetiapine (Seroquel)	_____ _____ _____ _____ (especially of the face/tongue/throat), severe dizziness, trouble breathing; immediate medical attention is required
Central nervous system stimulants	Amphetamine, dextroamphetamine _____, methylphenidate _____	_____ _____
Sedatives	Eszopiclone _____	_____

MEDICATIONS USED TO TREAT DIABETES

Describe diabetes:

_____

_____

_____

MEDICATION USED TO TREAT BACTERIAL, VIRAL, AND FUNGAL INFECTIONS

Answer the following questions.

1. What does MRSA stand for? _____

2. What three pathogens can most skin infections be attributed to? _____

_____

3. What skin reactions can be caused by antibiotics? _____

_____

_____

4. Describe a virus: _____

_____

5. List the skin conditions caused by antivirals: _____

_____

_____

6. What is a pathogenic fungus? _____

_____

7. Give an example of superficial mycoses: _____

8. List the skin conditions that oral antifungals can cause: _____

_____

MEDICATIONS USED TO TREAT BONE DISEASES

Answer the following questions.

1. Which ethnic groups' members are more susceptible to osteoporosis? _____

_____

2. What skin effects do rheumatoid arthritis drugs cause? _____

_____

_____

_____

3. How do corticosteroids function? _____

_____

_____

4. What skin effects do corticosteroids have? _____

_____

_____

_____

MEDICATIONS USED FOR PAIN MANAGEMENT

Fill in the information that is missing from the chart.

Classification	Medication Examples	Skin Side Effects
Narcotic analgesics	Codeine, fentanyl transdermal patch (Duragesic), hydrocodone (Vicodin), hydromorphone (Dilaudid), meperidine (Demerol), morphine (MS Contin), nalbuphine (Nubain), oxycodone (OxyContin), oxymorphone (Opana), propoxyphene (Darvon)	_____ _____ _____ _____
Nonsteroidal anti-inflammatory agents (NSAIDs)	Celecoxib (Celebrex), diflunisal (Dolobid), etodolac (Lodine), fenoprofen (Nalfon), flurbiprofen (Ocufen), ibuprofen (Advil, Motrin), ketoprofen (Rhodis), meloxicam (Mobic)	_____ _____
Nonnarcotic analgesics	Acetaminophen, salicylates (aspirin)	_____ _____
Muscle relaxants	Chlorzoxazone (Parafon-Forte), dantrolene (Dantrium), methocarbamol (Robaxin)	_____ _____ _____ _____ _____

Date: _____3/23/22_____

Rating: _____

TREATMENT VARIATIONS

Describe the purpose for each step. Then, write these steps on a 3"× 5" card for future reference.

1. Cleanse: All treatments start with removal of a client's makeup and then a complete facial cleansing

2. Tone: To balance, hydrate or soothe clients skin.

3. Water/moisture: Can be administer it using a steamer, compress, Help attract moisture from the treatment.

4. Exfoliation: Soften the skin for gentler and easier exfoliation and to keep an exfoliating agent

5. Massage: For gentle effeurage or very light tapotement

6. Extraction: Generally should be done after the skin is warmed, softened, and hydrated.

7. Mask: Can be done with a soft setting creams or gels, drying and exfoliating clays.

8. Penetration of ampoules or treatment serums: *Depending on the clients needs treatment may include machines such as ultrasand or microcurrent.*

9. Protection (moisturization and SPF): *Protects the skin from environmental insults including the sun.*

FOR DEHYDRATED SKIN

Fill in the missing steps for a facial for dehydrated skin.

1. Cleanse.

2. *Tone*

3. Use hydrating ampoule with steam.

4. *While still steaming, massage to help the ampule*

5. *Tone*

6. Exfoliate.

7. Tone.

8. *Use penetrating serums or ampoules*

9. *Massage*

10. Use hydrating mask.

11. *Tone*

12. Apply protection.

FOR CLOGGED SKIN

Fill in the missing steps for a facial for clogged resistive skin.

1. Cleanse the skin thoroughly. Do not apply toner to the skin until after extraction as toner will constrict pores, making extraction more difficult.

2. Apply desincrustant to soften hardened sebaceous impactions.

3. Apply steam. If desired penetrate the desincrustant product with negative galvanic current.

4. *Penetrate the disincrustant product with negative galavinc*

5. Gently extract.

6. _Apply toner_

7. If the skin is not too clogged, apply a non-oily hydration fluid and massage gently.

8. _Apply clay-based mask_

9. Apply protection.

FOR SENSITIVE SKIN

Fill in the missing steps for a facial for sensitive skin.

1. _Cleanse with gentle effleurage_

2. Apply gentle toner.

3. Use soothing serum with cool steam or moisture.

4. _____

5. Use penetrating soothing serums or ampoules. This may be followed with application of cool cryo-globes or mild iontophoresis, if appropriate.

6. _Apply a calming gel mask_

7. Apply protection.

THERMOTHERAPY: HEAT AND COOL MODALITIES

Answer the following questions.

1. Explain three ways to apply thermotherapy:

   a. _Heated steam_

   b. _Stones_

   c. _Wet towels_

2. Explain four ways to cool the skin:

   a. _Lucas spray_

   b. _cool steam_

   c. _cool stone_

   d. _cool towels_

3. How can you apply pressure therapy? _Warm stone on a muscle_

4. What is the benefit of applying a refrigerator-cold towel? _Help soothe and reduce redness_

THERMOTHERAPY FOR CLOGGED PORES

Fill in the missing steps for a facial using thermotherapy for clogged pores.

1. Prepare the client for treatment.

2. Cleanse. Moisten the skin using warm cotton compresses or sponges.

    a. Apply a cleanser suitable to remove makeup with your gloved hands.

    b. Massage the cleanser to loosen makeup.

    c. Remove the cleanser using warm cloth, sponges, or compresses.

3. Analysis and consultation.

    a. Place moistened eye pads on eyes.

    b. Examine the client's skin under magnifying lamp. Observe for the level of sensitivity and skin response to cleansing. Confirm that the selected products and that the temperature changes planned will be appropriate.

4. _Apply a serum designed to loosen impactions._

5. _____.

    a. Use an enzyme exfoliant following manufacturer's guidelines. Wrap the face in two hot towels in a classical barber wrap. The towel should be very warm but comfortable. Place the second towel on top of the first.

    b. Leave the towel on the skin approximately 8 to 10 minutes. If the towel cools too quickly, use steam to keep it warm or replace the top towel with a fresh one.

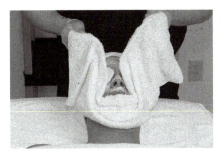

    c. Remove top towel.

    d. Use the lower towel to remove enzyme from the skin.

6. Extraction. Before starting, refresh gloves if necessary.

    a. Apply a pre-extraction serum if desired. Follow manufacturer's guidelines.

    b. Use cotton swab technique or comedone extractor to perform extraction.

    c. If skin begins to welt, redden severely, or swell, stop extraction immediately.

    d. Limit the extraction to 5 to 10 minutes only, particularly during the first visit.

7. Wipe the skin with a soothing or antiseptic toner.

8. _____

    (a.) Apply soothing serum.

    b. Apply cool wet towels wrapping the face in classical barber wrap. As an alternative, you can use cold globes over gauze, slowly stroking across the entire face, one area at a time.

    c. Allow the skin to calm about 10 minutes.

    d. Remove towels.

9. _Apply a hydrating fluid and sunscreen_

10. Advise client to treat any extracted area carefully and avoid touching it. Advise the client not to apply makeup for at least two hours.

11. _Remind client to avoid sun_

12. _Determine client appropriate home care products_

13. Follow cleanup and disinfection in accordance with state regulations.

14. _Reset room and prepare for next client_

15. Now use a 3 × 5 card and create a treatment guide for this skin issue.

ROSACEA AND SENSITIVE SKIN TREATMENTS

List four concepts for sensitive skin.

1. _Use products that support the barrier function_

2. _Avoid materials, products, or procedures that irritate the skin_

3. _Use products designed for sensitive skin_

4. _Incorporate products with ingredients that have been shown to decrease sensitivity._

TREATMENT CONTRAINDICATIONS FOR TREATING SENSITIVE SKIN

For each statement about treating sensitive skin, write T for True or F for False.

1. __T__ Waxing should be avoided on sensitive skin.

2. __F__ Always use a high pH exfoliation chemical.

3. __F__ Perform a prolonged massage.

4. __T__ Avoid overdrying masks or leaving clay masks on too long.

5. __T__ Avoid heat exposure.

6. __F__ Microdermabrasion can be done for all clients that have sensitive skin.

7. __T__ Avoid paraffin.

8. __F__ Extractions can be done for a prolonged amount of time.

9. __T__ Avoid using products containing isopropyl or SD alcohol.

10. __T__ Avoid heavily mentholated or alcohol-based treatment products.

11. __T__ Use non-fragranced products.

TREATMENT FOR SENSITIVE SKIN

Fill in the missing steps for a facial for sensitive skin.

1. Cleanse. Dampen the skin using cool (not cold), wet cotton compresses.

   a. Apply a gentle, non-fragranced cleanser with your gloved hands.

   b. Gently massage the cleanser using light effleurage.

   c. Remove the cleanser using cool, wet cotton pads.

2. __Place moistered eye pads on eyes__

   a. Place moistened eye pads on eyes.

   b. Examine skin under magnifying lamp. Observe for level of sensitivity and skin response to cleansing. Confirm that selected products will be appropriate.

3. Apply a lightweight, non-fragranced hydrating fluid designed for sensitive skin to the face.

   a. If you use warm steam, place steamer head at a distance of 18 to 20 inches from the face and use for only a few minutes.

   b. Cool steam, if available, is preferable.

4. _Use a gentle enzyme exfoliant following the manufacture_

5. _Remove the exfoliant with lukewarm towels_

6. Spray the skin with a mild, non-fragranced, non-alcohol toner.

7. Calm. If the skin is still very red after extraction, apply cool, wet compresses for about five minutes. Do *not* apply any product.

8. _Apply hydrating fluid/serum_

9. Mask.

10. _Apply a gentle, nonfragranced hydrating fluid and sunscreen_

11. Now create a 3 × 5 card with skin treatment steps for this skin condition.

CLIENT REACTIONS IN THE TREATMENT ROOM

Answer the following questions.

1. List some negative reactions that a client could have in the treatment room. _Client may have a stinging or burning reaction._

2. What should be done if a client has a negative reaction? _Remove whatever is on the client face. Apply cool wet compress_

3. What are two examples of retinoids? _Tretinoin and Tazarotene_

4. What is a normal side effect of using retinoids? _Redness and peeling_

5. What should be avoided for someone who is on retinoids? _Scented and Fragranced products, Alcohol-based lotions, Stripping products, abrasive BHA. Do not wax._

MANUAL MICRODERMABRASION

Fill in the missing steps for a facial using manual microdermabrasion.

1. Wash and disinfect hands.

2. _Cleanse_

3. _Remove face makeup with cleansing lotion_

4. Massage. Perform massage as usual for your treatment.

5. _Apply microderm product and perform treatment_

6. Tone.

7. Treat and mask as appropriate for client's skin to conclude the treatment. Apply serum(s) appropriate for client's skin.

8. _Apply additional serum and sun protection._

ENZYMES

Answer the following questions.

1. Enzymes are a proteolytic, which means they are _dissolving_

2. Enzyme peels are suitable for the following conditions:

   a. _Oily and clogged skin_

   b. _Dry or dehydrated skin with cell buildup_

   c. _Dull or lifeless looking skin with tremendous buildup of dead cells_

   d. _Skin with multiple milia_

   e. _Clients who desire a smoother appreance to their skin_

ACIDS

Answer the following questions.

1. List the characteristics of alpha hydroxy acids:

   a. _____

   b. _____

   c. _____

   d. _____

2. What is a beta hydroxy acid attracted to? _____

3. What is the highest strength of glycolic acid that the Cosmetic Ingredient Review committee recommends estheticians use? _____

4. How does an acid peel help a client with strengthening his or her skin's elasticity? _____
   _____
   _____

5. Why is it important for a client to use products with alpha hydroxy acids prior to receiving a peel? _____

ALPHA HYDROXY ACID EXFOLIATIONS

Fill in the missing steps for a facial using exfoliating acids.

1. Cleanse the skin with makeup-removing cleanser.

2. _____

3. _____

4. Protection of sensitive tissue.

5. _____

6. _____

PRECAUTIONS FOR AHA EXFOLIATIONS

For each statement, write a T for True and an F for False.

1. _____ Always make sure the skin has been pretreated with lower-strength alpha hydroxy acid at home for at least two weeks before administering a 30 percent AHA treatment.

2. _____ After waxing, wait at least 24 hours before performing an AHA treatment.

3. _____ It is permissible to perform an AHA treatment on anyone with a skin disorder.

4. _____ Do not use the peeling agent on a male client immediately after he has shaved.

5. _____ Accutane patients can receive AHA treatments.

6. _____ Do not use AHAs on someone who is using keratolytics.

7. _____ If the skin is irritated, it is permissible to use AHAs.

8. _____ If the client has a history of herpes simplex, refer him or her to a doctor.

9. _____ Clients do not have to wear sunscreen after receiving an AHA treatment.

10. _____ Check with a client to see how his or her skin has reacted in past treatments (if any).

TREATMENTS FOR HYPERPIGMENTED SKIN AND SUPERFICIAL PEELS

Answer the following questions.

1. Treatments for hyperpigmented skin can include: _____

_____

2. Most experienced professionals agree that TCA belongs in the hands of dermatologists and _____.

3. A very superficial or superficial peel removes cells from the _____ only.

4. An example of a superficial peel is a _____.

5. What type of clients should not have stronger superficial chemical peeling performed?

a. _____

b. _____

c. _____

_____

_____

6. The following clients should have written permission from a physician to receive a chemical peeling treatment.

a. _____

b. _____

c. _____

d. _____

_____

7. What are the benefits of a superficial peel? _____

_____

_____

JESSNER'S SOLUTION OR 20 PERCENT BHA TREATMENT

Fill in the missing steps for a facial using chemical peels.

1. Complete the pre-exfoliation consultation procedure.

2. _____

3. _____

4. Put on gloves.

5. Perform a second cleansing.

6. _____

7. Follow manufacturer's directions for application of occlusive barrier to corners of the mouth and nose and around the eyes.

8. _____

9. Apply the liquid solution on the face.

10. Place a small fan so that it blows gently on the client's face.

11. _____

12. Following the manufacturer's directions, rinse frost and residue from the skin using a neutralizer as recommended.

13. _____

MASK THERAPIES

Fill in the chart below.

Suffocation	Triggering increased circulation to the area
_____	Adding moisture
_____	Purging, drawing, absorption of impurities
_____	Soothing
_____	Rejuvenating
_____	Smoothing the skin

APPLICATION OF A POWDER MASK

Fill in the missing steps for applying a powder mask.

1. Apply appropriate serums for the skin.

2. Apply a layer of moisturizer to skin.

3. _____

4. _____

5. Apply damp cotton rounds to protect the eye area.

6. Apply a single-layer gauze sheet over the client's face to facilitate removal.

7. _____

8. _____

9. Remove the mask by placing your fingers along the hairline perimeter of mask just above jaw level.

10. _____

11. Apply sun protection.

Activity: Create a reference sheet from your facility's back bar products by skin conditions. Review your selection with your instructor to ensure you have appropriate products.

	Dehy-drated Skin	Clogged Skin	Sensi-tive	Theromo-therapy Clogged Pores	Manual Micro D	AHA	BHA	Hyper-Pigment-ation Peel
Cleanser								
Toner								
Exfoliate								
Massage								
Mask								
Serum or Ampoule								
SPF								

17 Advanced Skin Care Massage

Date: _____

Rating: _____

ADVANCED FACIAL MOVEMENTS

Answer the following questions.

1. List a few of the specialty massages:

a. _____

b. _____

c. _____

2. List the nine contraindications for massage:

a. _____

b. _____

c. _____

d. _____

e. _____

f. _____

g. _____

h. _____

i. _____

3. What are the key components to a massage?

a. _____

b. _____

c. _____

SELECTING AND INCORPORATING ADVANCED FACIAL MOVEMENTS

Describe how to perform each of these massage techniques in your own words.

1. Center point: _____
_____
_____
_____

2. Sinus relief: _____
_____
_____
_____
_____
_____

3. Feather off: _____
_____

4. Forehead press: _____
_____

5. Gallop 1-2-1: _____
_____
_____
_____

6. Full face sweep: _____
_____

7. Rolling along: _____
_____
_____
_____

8. Feels good: _____
_____
_____
_____
_____

9. Décolleté sweep: _____
_____
_____
_____
_____

10. Ski up: _____

_____

11. Neck-shoulder-arm: _____

_____

_____

_____

_____

_____

12. Rock-a-bye: _____

_____

_____

ADVANCED BACK MOVEMENTS

List two advanced back movements.

1. _____

2. _____

SHIATSU MASSAGE FOR THE FACE

Each touch in Shiatsu is performed to the count of three. List the three items.

1. _____

2. _____

3. _____

When performing Shiatsu, it is important to remember the following.

1. _____

_____

_____

_____

2. _____

_____

_____

3. _____

4. _____

_____

_____

_____

PROCEDURE FOR THE SHIATSU MASSAGE FOR HEAD AND NECK

Fill in the missing steps.

Preparation

1. Set up the facial lounge and prepare the room for the client.

2. Decant massage vehicle (optional).

3. Before the client gets onto the lounge, allow him or her to put on a gown.

4. _____

Procedure

5. _____

6. Glide your hands up over the face to the forehead.

7. Begin at the top of the head, running your fingers through the hair.

8. Running Water

Gently brushing the scalp, run your fingertips from the hairline back through the client's hair.

9. Taking a small section of hair, gently pull small sections of hair, one at a time, all over the client's head.

10. _____

_____

_____

11. _____

_____

a. Move your thumbs to the center of the forehead and repeat.

b. _____

_____

c. _____

_____

12. Move your hands to the inner corner of the eye and, with your thumbs, gently press the inner corner of the eye sockets for three to four seconds.

13. _____

14. With the finger and thumb, gently pinch across the length of the brow.

15. Placing your thumbs at the outer ends of the eyebrows, gently press the bony ridge and ends of the brows.

16. _____
    _____

17. Glide your thumbs to the sides of the nose.

18. Gently apply pressure with your thumbs, starting at the sides of the nose, moving in half-inch (1.3-cm) steps along the top of the zygomatic arch toward the temples.

19. Glide back to sides of nose. Repeat this pattern, from the corners of the nose back just under the zygomatic bone toward the ears.

20. From the ears, glide in a straight line down to masseter muscle. Apply light pressure at the center of the masseter muscle and release.

21. _____
    _____

22. _____

23. Cup the chin with your hands, using your thumbs in the chin groove below the lower lip.

24. Press along the center of the chin. Moving to the hollow at the jaw, press and release.

25. With thumbs still at the jaw hollows, lay the side of small fingers in the hollows under the jawline.

26. Glide along the hollow of the jaw back toward the ears.

27. At the ears, roll your hands (using the pads at the base of your thumbs) in and down the side of the neck and off the client.

REFLEXOLOGY

Answer the following question.

1. Explain reflexology: _____
    _____
    _____
    _____

STONES MASSAGE TECHNIQUES

Answer the following questions.

1. Explain warm stone massage: _____

_____

_____

2. How would cold stones be beneficial? _____

_____

STONES MASSAGE PROCEDURE

Fill in the missing steps in the procedure for stone massage for face.

Preparation

1. Set up the facial lounge in the typical manner and prepare the treatment room for client.

2. Gather supplies for the facial treatment.

3. _____

4. Turn on the stone warming unit and heat following manufacturer's guidelines. Ensure that the heat of the the stones does not exceed 120°F (49°C).

5. Perform all massage steps of the facial before starting the stone massage. Apply massage vehicle.

6. _____

7. Turn on the steamer if you choose to use it during the massage.

Procedure

8. _____

9. _____

_____

10. When stones feel comfortable to handle, test one against the client's skin to assure that the temperature is comfortable for the client.

11. Start at the corrigator with one stone held between the thumb and first finger of each hand. All movements are gliding, alternating hands and using stroking movements, unless otherwise specified.

12. _____

13. _____

_____

14. _____

15. _____

16. _____

17. _____

18. Glide stones along the perimeter of the face to meet at the center of the chin.

19. _____

20. Simultaneously perform circles, moving from the chin along the jawline to the ears.

21. Glide back to the chin.

22. Using both hands simultaneously, glide up and repeat this process in the hollow above the jawline along the lower teeth moving from the chin to the ears.

23. Glide back to the corners of the mouth.

24. _____

25. _____

26. Using alternating hands, perform strokes from the corners of the nose, across the cheeks, and back toward the temples, starting on the right side of the nose.

27. Repeat on the left side of the face.

28. Repeat steps 12 through 14 three times, and then glide your hands to the temples.

29. _____

_____

30. _____

31. _____

32. _____

33. Moving both hands simultaneously, glide from the top of the nose up over the brow. Continue gliding to the temples.

34. Continue gliding to the jawline.

35. Continue down the side of the neck and bring your left hand to join your right hand at the collarbone below the right ear, all in one continuous movement.

36. Alternating hands, stroke up the neck to jawline, starting on the right side of the face.

37. Repeat movements across the neck.

38. Finish with strokes up the left side of the neck under the ears.

39. _____
_____

40. _____

41. From the temple on the right side, continue feathering strokes to the hairline. Repeat feathering strokes across the width of the forehead.

42. _____
_____

43. _____
_____

44. _____
_____

45 Glide stones so each hand is positioned at the base of each ear.

46. _____
_____

47. Finish by stroking stones simultaneously off each shoulder.

LYMPHATIC MASSAGE FOR THE FACE AND NECK

Fill in the blanks using the word bank below.

bruising	lymph
healing crisis	lymph nodes
infections	lymphocytes
injury	skillfully directed touch

1. Disease-causing organisms easily enter the body via the mouth, nose, and eyes, and the body's immune system, including the _____ of the head and neck, needs to respond.

2. Lymph drainage massage stimulates the circulation of lymph and _____ through the facial and cervical lymph nodes.

3. LDM to the face and neck effectively reduces _____ and edema following injury or surgery, including dental and cosmetic surgery.

4. Facial edema can be due to allergies, hormones, medication, fatigue, illness, infection, _____ , excess salt in the diet, and weeping.

5. LDM stimulates a sluggish immune system to more activity by increasing the circulation of _____ and _____ .

6. Although LDM is focused on superficial tissues, the muscles underneath also respond to light _____ and will relax.

7. Many people have chronically swollen lymph nodes, often from repeated _____ and childhood illness.

8. A _____ means simply that the client might experience a flare-up of old symptoms.

9. Unscramble the following names of the lymph nodes.

ucularria   _____

stnmubeal   _____

msibdarunbula   _____

ntraerio viccealr naihc   _____

rioportse relvciac hinac   _____

PROCEDURE FOR MANUAL LYMPH DRAINAGE MASSAGE

Fill in the missing steps in the procedure for LDM for the neck.

Preparation

1. Set up the facial lounge and treatment room.

2 Gather supplies.

3. Consult with the client to ensure that there are no contraindications to treatment and to complete all intake forms.

4. Ensure that the client has signed informed consent to service.

5. _____

6. Offer a bolster if the client needs one under his or her knees.

Procedure

This treatment is done in two phases—first the neck and then the face.

7. Sit or stand at the client's head.

8. Apply skin-cleansing agent.

9. _____
_____

10. As the towel cools, massage gently through the towel to relax the tissues. Before removing the towel, use it to gently wipe the face.

11. _____
_____

12. _____
_____
_____

13. Place your fingertips along the anterior/medial edge of the sternocleidomastoid muscles and massage very lightly, using just enough pressure to move the skin, for at least a minute.

14. Place your fingertips along the lateral/posterior edges of the sternocleidomastoid muscles and massage for at least a minute.

15. Massage the postauricularnodes, between the ears and the mastoid process, posterior and inferior to the ears. Use three or four fingers, flat against the skin, to stretch the skin gently in a circular direction, counting each circle carefully to keep the pace very slow. Massage for at least a minute.

16. Slide the flat pads of fingers of both hands under the neck, covering the skin from the bottom of the neck and hairline. Perform seven stationary circles, moving the skin on the back of the neck over the cervical vertebrae, taking about a minute to complete the seven circles.

17. _____
_____

18. Place two flat fingers inside the triangle bordered by the sternocleidomastoid muscle, the clavicle, and the scalene muscles, and again perform stationary circles for a full minute.

19. _____
_____

20. _____

_____

Caution: Omit Steps 21, 22, and 23 (the front of the neck) for any client who has thyroid abnormalities.

21. Place flat fingertips in the depression between the thyroid cartilage and the sternocleidomastoid muscles, and perform rotary massage using very light pressure.

22. _____

_____

23. Use effleurage movements on the throat and the back of the neck. The direction of pressure follows lymph drainage.

CHAPTER 18 Advanced Facial Devices

Date: _____

Rating: _____

INTRODUCTION

Look for the following terms in the word search puzzle below.

LED devices	IPL	photodynamic	ultrasonic
skin analysis devices	electrodessication	microcurrent	

```
A  D  A  J  V  D  A  U  J  I  U  Z  K  P  T  L  G  S  T  N
O  O  C  N  F  P  H  L  P  E  Y  G  Y  U  N  L  Y  Z  S  H
R  S  V  C  A  Z  W  T  O  L  B  M  O  W  D  D  Z  K  I  B
X  N  K  V  S  M  J  R  P  E  Y  G  O  D  B  X  I  F  G  K
X  K  W  W  E  H  C  A  M  C  O  Z  F  T  K  N  R  L  T  M
E  K  Q  Z  R  E  L  S  Y  T  E  L  N  K  A  M  S  N  L  U
S  X  Y  L  H  V  H  O  E  R  Y  M  T  N  Y  N  E  P  F  A
P  C  B  B  D  O  R  N  B  O  I  Y  A  B  W  R  I  C  L  W
I  U  J  I  A  G  A  I  R  D  O  L  C  H  R  M  I  C  W  L
C  Z  H  L  U  K  A  C  Y  E  Y  J  L  U  O  M  D  H  U  H
L  E  D  D  E  V  I  C  E  S  C  B  C  U  A  U  P  Y  N  L
X  F  F  N  P  I  J  W  I  S  X  O  E  N  L  W  K  A  K  H
S  P  L  L  Z  R  K  S  T  I  R  A  Y  V  S  U  N  F  Z  C
Q  Y  Z  L  G  W  D  V  X  C  D  D  Q  L  S  W  L  X  X  B
N  K  C  I  V  E  V  V  I  A  O  W  M  E  K  V  K  A  V  H
I  I  A  P  V  Y  C  M  V  T  D  C  U  U  J  M  L  L  J  W
B  Z  Q  I  P  U  X  L  O  I  W  V  A  X  B  Q  G  V  I  R
H  U  C  W  H  K  Y  H  M  O  R  R  I  D  B  Q  V  C  C  E
O  E  K  H  K  G  P  C  A  N  I  T  U  R  O  A  L  O  O  D
S  W  E  Q  Q  W  M  B  G  U  B  J  Q  W  F  L  S  Q  S  K
```

THE PURCHASING PROCESS

Answer the following questions.

1. An esthetician wanting to perform specific services needs to contact his or her
_____ to determine if they are within his or her scope of practice.

2. List what you would consider when analyzing your practice's needs:

   a. _____

   b. _____

   c. _____

   d. _____

3. In your own words, state how you would research the best manufacturer.
_____
_____

4. What should you consider for maintenance? _____
_____
_____
_____

5. What should you consider when it comes to disposable/reusable parts?
_____
_____
_____

6. What forms of training might a manufacturer offer? _____
_____

7. What types of labels would be on various machines? _____
_____

IPL FACIAL REJUVENATION

Answer the following questions.

1. Explain the research by Patrick Bitters, M.D. _____
_____
_____
_____

2. Explain the research by Robert Weiss, M.D. _____
_____
_____

_____

_____

_____

_____

FACIAL REJUVENATION

Answer the following questions.

1. Describe photorejuvenation:

_____

_____

2. IPL facial rejuvenation has become the gold standard due to the _____, noncoherent, _____ flashlamp effects.

3. During the procedure, intense white light is pulsed with wavelengths ranging from _____ in the energy spectrum.

4. List the common conditions that can be treated with IPL device for photorejuvenation:

   a. _____

   b. _____

   c. _____

   d. _____

   e. _____

   f. _____

   g. _____

THE CONSULTATION

Answer the following questions.

1. What are some medical issues that you need to ask a client about during the consultation on the client intake form?

   a. _____

   b. _____

   c. _____

   d. _____

e. _____

f. _____

g. _____

h. _____

i. _____

j. _____

k. _____

l. _____

m. _____

2. What tool should you use to evaluate a client's skin type? _____

_____

3. List examples of "red flag" clients:

a. _____

_____

b. _____

c. _____

_____

d. _____

_____

e. _____

_____

4. Name some antibiotics that can be photosensitizing:

a. _____

b. _____

c. _____

5. List the possible contraindications to treatment:

a. _____

b. _____

c. _____

d. _____

e. _____

_____

f. _____

g. _____

h. _____

i. _____

j. _____

k. _____

IPL PHOTOREJUVENATION

Unscramble the names of the following implements and materials used in an IPL photorejuvenation procedure.

resncale   _____

eiltcn rpead   _____

lge olconat   _____

uns roetpiotnc   _____

rewta wolb   _____

rneot   _____

tops-retatnetm mures   _____

evlogs   _____

eldssibaop pogsens   _____

rottviepce weyaere   _____

avaltinoeu msrof   _____

Fill in the missing steps in the following procedure.

Preparation

1. Prepare treatment lounge and client gown.

2. Assemble towels and disposables.

3. Set up products and protective devices.

4. Have ready the appropriate sign for the outside door.

5. Have client cleanse his or her face in a separate waiting area and apply topical anesthetic on the treatment site as directed and needed for the specific device. (Some devices require no anesthetics.) The client's face is to be cleansed, and if topical anesthesia is used it should be applied with time for absorption before treatment. Some treatments require no anesthetics.

6. Review client post-care instructions. These can be discussed while any anesthetics absorb.

7. _____

8. Hang up the appropriate eyewear on the door for staff members who may enter.

9. Turn on the IPL machine. _____

10. _____

11. Replace any IPL handpieces and filters that need replacing.

Procedure

12. Secure client's hair away from the face.

13. _____

14. _____

15. Ask if the client has tanned recently or used self-tanner within the past month.

16. Reconfirm areas of treatment and the client's goals.

17. Take documentary photographs.

18. Enter the client's demographic data into the IPL system, if required by device.

19. _____
_____

20. Double-check all parameters before treating.

21. _____

22. Put on gloves.

23. _____

24. _____

25. Float the filter in the gel if this is appropriate for your specific device. The degree of floating in the gel will vary based on the type of device and if the filter has a chilled sapphire window.

26. After testing the spot on the side of the face, assess clinical end points.

    a. Observe for slight erythema.

    b. Observe for darkening of a vessel or vasospasm.

    c. Observe for darkening or redness of a lentigo.

27. If the test response is acceptable, continue treatment with the same settings. If not, raise or lower the joules accordingly or switch to a different parameter or filter.

28. Start treatment with the forehead. Be careful of hair line and eyebrows. Protect them with tongue depressor.

29. _____

_____

30. Place the handpiece perpendicular to the skin and floating in the gel, if one is required by the manufacturer.

31. Fire trigger.

32. _____

33. _____

34. _____

35. _____

36. Move to the nose, upper lip, and chin in a systematic manner. Then move to below and above the lips, being careful not to work over lip vermillion.

37. Progress to the cheeks and treat across the cheeks in a systematic manner.

38. Remove any residual gel.

39. _____

40. Apply soothing agent and protective sunscreen.

Post-procedure

41. Supply the client with an ice pack, if recommended or needed.

42. _____

_____

43. _____

_____

44. Complete the documentation on the procedure and place photos in client's file.

Cleanup and Disinfection

45. Turn off machine with the key following manufacturer guidelines.

46. Wipe down the machine with germicidal wipes.

47. _____

48. _____

49. Reset and prepare the room for the next client.

50. _____
_____

LASER AND IPL HAIR REMOVAL

Fill in the chart below.

Lasers and Their Efficacy in Hair Removal

Laser Or Light	Skin Type	Hair Color	Type Of Hair
Pulsed diode	I–IV	_____	Coarse
Ruby	_____	_____	Fine and coarse
Normal mode Nd:YAG	_____	_____	_____
Q-Switch Nd:YAG	I–VI (temporary removal only)	_____	_____
Alexandrite	_____	_____	Fine and coarse
Intense pulsed light	I–IV	Black to light brown	_____

INTENSE PULSED LIGHT

Fill in the blanks using terms from the word bank below.

1,000 nm	pigment
hair reduction	polychromatic
nonablative	

1. Intense pulsed light is _____ and broadband.

2. The wavelength on an intense pulsed light is between 400 nm to _____.

3. The filters that are used create wavelengths that selectively target different skin structures—hair, _____ , or vessels.

4. Some IPL devices have demonstrated efficiency in _____

5. IPL treatments are gaining in popularity because they _____, more comfortable, faster, and less expensive for both the client and the practitioner.

6. List the benefits of laser or IPL hair removal versus other treatment modalities:

a. _____

b. _____

c. _____
_____

d. _____
_____

e. _____

f. _____

7. List the drawbacks of laser or IPL hair removal versus other treatment modalities:

a. _____

b. _____

c. _____

d. _____

e. _____

f. _____

g. _____

h. _____

8. List four safety guidelines for the laser room:

a. _____

b. _____

c. _____

d. _____

9. List five safety guidelines for the technician in the laser room.

a. _____

b. _____

c. _____

d. _____

e. _____

10. What are the four main categories of excess hair growth?

a. _____

b. _____

c. _____

d. _____

11. What is hypertrichosis? _____

12. What is hirsutism? _____
_____

13. What is a hair-bearing flap? _____
_____

14. What is a cosmetic reason for wanting hair removal? _____
_____

15. What is the most important conversation you can have with your client? _____
_____
_____

16. What are the contraindications for laser hair removal?_____
_____
_____
_____

Fill in the chart below.

Skin Type and Laser Hair Removal

Fitzpatrick Skin Type	Description	Laser Hair Removal Considerations
Type I	Very fair skin accompanied by blond or light-red hair and blue or green eyes; never tans, always burns	_____ _____ _____
Type II	Fair skin accompanied by light-brown or red hair and green, blue, or brown eyes. Occasionally tans, always burns.	_____ _____
Type III	Medium skin accompanied by brown hair and brown eyes; _____	_____ _____
Type IV	Olive skin, accompanied by brown or black hair and dark-brown or black eyes; always tans, rarely burns	_____ _____ _____
Type V	Dark-brown skin accompanied by black hair and black eyes; _____	_____ _____ _____ _____ _____
Type VI	Black skin accompanied by black hair and black eyes; _____	_____ _____ _____ _____ _____

THE CONSULATION

1. List the important information to discuss with a client before a laser hair removal treatment:

a. _____

b. _____

c. _____

d. _____

e. _____

f. _____

g. _____

h. _____

2. List the steps to complete prior to treatment:

a. _____
_____

b. _____

c. _____

d. _____

e. _____

f. _____

LASER HAIR REMOVAL TREATMENT

Answer the following questions.

1. What is a drawback of using a topical anesthesic? _____
_____
_____
_____

2. What are the technical issues that affect the overall result of the hair removal process?
_____
_____

3. How can the skin be cooled during the treatments? _____

4. What is the spot size?_____
_____

5. Describe wavelength: _____
_____
_____

6. How is energy fluence measured? _____

7. What does thermal storage coefficient mean? _____

8. What is the pulse duration (or pulse width)? _____

_____

9. Describe thermal relaxation time: _____

_____

10. List the home-care directions:

a. _____

_____

b. _____

_____

c. _____

_____

d. _____

_____

_____

e. _____

_____

_____

_____

f. _____

_____

_____

_____

g. _____

_____

_____

h. _____

_____

i. _____

_____

11. List the treatment consequences of laser hair removal:

a. _____

_____

b. _____

_____

c. _____

12. Complications of laser hair removal include:

a. _____

b. _____

c. _____

d. _____

e. _____

13. How do you minimize liability concerns? _____

_____

PROCEDURE PERFORMING LASER OR IPL HAIR REMOVAL TREATMENT

Fill in the missing steps in the laser hair removal procedure

1. Unlock the laser device.

2. _____

3. _____

4. Set the treatment parameters according to manufacturer's guidelines or charted settings from previous treatment for the area, hair, and skin according to the response at the test site.

5. _____

_____

_____

_____

6. Compress the skin firmly with the handpiece to disperse the oxyhemoglobin (a chromophore that competes with melanin) away from the treatment area. Doing so allows for greater absorption of the laser light and reduces the risk of epidermal damage, as well as maneuvers the dermal papilla closer to the surface, which makes for a more effective treatment.

7. _____

8. _____

_____

9. _____

_____

_____

_____

_____

10. Read the skin. If topical anesthesia and cooling remedies have not reduced the client's discomfort, make adjustments.

11. _____

12. After treating the entire area, wipe down the skin with soothing antiseptic lotion.

LIGHT-EMITTING DIODES (LEDS)

Answer the following questions.

1. Explain a service using an LED device:

_____

_____

_____

_____

_____

2. What can be treated with the LED device?

a. _____

b. _____

c. _____

d. _____

e. _____

3. What are the contraindications to an LED treatment?

a. _____

b. _____

c. _____

d. _____

e. _____

f. _____

PHOTODYNAMIC THERAPY

Answer the following questions.

1. Photodynamic therapy is used with a photosensitizing drug enhancer called

   _____ .

2. What is this treatment used for?_____

3. How is this procedure performed? _____

   _____

   _____

   _____

MACHINE-AIDED MICRODERMABRASION

Answer the following questions.

1. When was microdermabrasion introduced to the U.S. market? _____

2. What has microdermabrasion been documented to help with?

   a. _____

   b. _____

   c. _____

3. Explain the various types of machines:

   a. Aluminum oxide crystals:

   _____

   _____

   _____

   _____

   b. Organic crystals:

   _____

   _____

   _____

   _____

   _____

   _____

   _____

   _____

   _____

   _____

c. Non-crystal devices:

_____
_____
_____
_____
_____
_____
_____

d. Vibrating ultrasonic paddles:

_____
_____
_____
_____

4. List some of the skin problems that microdermabrasion may help:

a. _____

b. _____
   _____

c. _____

d. _____

e. _____

5. List possible contraindications:

a. _____

b. _____

c. _____

d. _____

e. _____

f. _____

g. _____

h. _____

i. _____

MICRODERMABRASION PROCEDURE

Fill in the missing steps for a microdermabrasion procedure.

1. Position the client comfortably in a relaxing, reclining position with hair protected.

2. Make sure the client has removed all facial piercings, jewelry, and contact lenses.

3. _____

4. _____

5. Dry the skin.

6. Protect client's eyes with occlusive adhesive eyewear, pads, or moistened gauze.

7. _____

8. Follow manufacturer's recommendations for pressure settings, time exposure, and treatment protocol.

9. _____

   a. Skin should be slightly pink and comfortable.

   b. Using the medical pain response scale of 1 to 10 with 1 being no pain and 10 being the worst imaginable, client's response should never be higher than 5. Settings of 2 to 4 are comfortable and safe.

   c. Start with settings low and increase as you determine how the client is tolerating the strokes.

10. _____
    _____
    _____

11. Make vertical strokes on the entire width of the forehead, starting at the center just above the eyebrow and working toward the hairline above the temple. As you reach the side of the forehead, tip the end of the device slightly, loosening pressure contact for a smooth release.

12. _____
    _____

13. Continue to work in rows up toward the hairline. Ensure that the pressure is comfortable for the client and appropriate for the skin type.

14. Repeat horizontal passes on the other side of the forehead.

15. Repeat vertical and horizontal passes on each cheek, working from the nose to jaw outward and from the orbital bone to the chin.

16. Repeat both sets of passes on the chin.

17. _____

18. _____

_____ Use the orbital bone as a guideline for how close to the eyes to go.

_____

_____

_____

NOTE:

A. _____

_____

B.   For devices that are non-particle or crystal, the strokes can be made from the outer eye area inward toward the nose. Continue on the other side.

19. If making passes on other parts of the body, follow these guidelines:

20. Neck should be hyperextended with passes in a vertical direction and a lower pressure than used on the face. Start at the neck and draw up.

21. For the decollete, start in the center of the chest and stroke outward, holding the skin taunt.

22. Client should make a fist prior to treatment of the hands to produce a taut skin surface.

23. Passes on the forearms should be made in vertical direction, taking note of bony areas and skin thickness and texture.

24. After completing all microdermabrasion, brush away any loose crystals.

25. Rinse the face to ensure that you have removed all crystals.

26. _____

27. Conclude the treatment with soothing serum or lotion and sun protection.

ULTRASONIC TECHNOLOGY

Answer the following questions.

1. What does ultrasonic technology use to clean out pores? _____

2. How is product penetration achieved? _____

_____

_____

3. What is another name for the peel modality?

_____

ULTRASONIC FACIAL

Fill in the missing steps of the following procedure.

Part I

1. Drape the client and secure hair away from the face.

2. Pre-cleanse and remove makeup using a water-based cleanser.

3. Adjust machine settings per manufacturer instructions and based on client skin type.

4. Apply cleanser, combined with a small trace of water for moisture, to the client's face in small circular motions, leaving that area slightly wet. Use a mild desincrustation fluid on severely oily and congested skin types.

5. Attach the wristband (if recommended by manufacturer) to the client and insert ear pads and eye pads for protection, if required by your state regulations.

6. _____
   _____
   _____

7. _____

8. Starting with the forehead, gently secure/stretch the skin to be treated between your thumb and pointer finger, just as when you perform a microdermabrasion treatment.

   a. Hold the ultrasonic blade at a 45-degree angle with the blade tip facing downward.

   b. Gently glide the handpiece across the skin surface in a light forward movement and using no pressure. The wand should almost float across the skin on the water or hydrator. It is the water and the vibration that do the work. A proper stroke will yield a fine forward arch of moisture droplets spraying from where the blade touches the skin.

   c. Increase or decrease intensity as indicated by the manufacturer.

9. _____
   _____

10. Move to the right cheek and repeat movements.

11. _____

12. Ask the client to hold his or her lips in a compressed "M" while you stroke across and downward from the nose toward the upper lip.

13. Stroke downward on the nose.

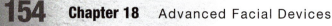

14. Use the corner of blade to stroke around the nasal flares.

15. _____

Part II

1. _____

2. _____

3. As in Part I, start with the forehead. If the skin shows signs of laxity, isolate areas in the same manner.

4. _____

5. _____
_____
_____

6. Increase or decrease intensity as indicated by the manufacturer.

7. _____

8. _____

9. Move to the cheeks, chin, and center of the face, repeating the process.

10. When you have treated the entire face, either move to the micro-amp phase of unit operations or conclude with a moisturizer and sun protection.

Part III

1. Some ultrasonic units have settings specifically for the microcurrent or homeostasis phase.

2. _____

3. _____

4. _____
_____

5. Rinse off excess gel with a warm, moist towel.

6. _____

7. Inform the client about appropriate home care.

8. _____

9. Perform cleanup and disinfection according to OSHA or your state's regulations.

10. _____

ELECTRODESSICATION DEVICES (RADIO FREQUENCY)

Answer the following questions.

1. What are electrodessication devices used for?

a. _____

b. _____

c. _____

d. _____

e. _____

f. _____

2. List contraindications for electrodessication:

a. _____

b. _____

c. _____

d. _____

e. _____

f. _____

g. _____

h. _____

i. _____

j. _____

MICROCURRENT "FACIAL TONING"

Answer the following questions.

1. What benefit can microcurrent offer? _____

2. What type of currents does microcurrent use? _____

3. What is the conductor for transferring the current? _____

INDICATIONS FOR TREATMENT

Fill in the blanks in the following chart.

Desired Treatment	Muscle Group	Technique
Reduction of eyelid hooding and brow drooping	Orbicularis oculi muscle closes the eyelid and compresses the lacrimal sac (tear duct)	Lifting, strengthening, and tightening
Reduction of jawline laxity and skin drooping	_____ _____ _____	_____ _____
Reduction of furrowing and lines between brows	_____ _____ _____	Relaxing and lengthening
Reduction of furrowing and lines between brows	_____ _____	_____
Reduction of forehead lines and laxity	_____ _____ _____	_____ _____
Reduction of marionette lines	Risorius muscle retracts the mouth	Lifting, strengthening, and tightening
Reduction of marionette lines	_____ _____ _____ _____	_____ _____

CONTRAINDICATIONS TO TREATMENT

What are the contraindications to microcurrent?

1. _____

2. _____

3. _____

4. _____

5. _____

6. _____

7. _____

8. _____

9. _____

MANAGEMENT OF COMPLICATIONS

Fill in the following chart.

Side Effect	Possible Interventions
Excessive swelling	_____ _____ _____
Excessive skin reaction	_____ _____ _____ _____ _____
Blistering or crusting	_____ _____ _____
Hyperpigmentation	_____ _____ _____
Hypopigmentation	_____
Infection	Physician may order antibiotic, antiviral, or antifungal medications.
Scarring	_____ _____ _____

19 Advanced Hair Removal

Date: _____

Rating: _____

SAFETY AND DISINFECTION FIRST

Answer the following questions.

1. During a hair removal procedure, when should you wear gloves?

   _____

   _____

2. If a client has a history of the herpes virus, what should the client do?

   _____

   _____

3. Genital warts are a viral infection caused by the human papilloma virus. If you see this condition on a client who comes in for a bikini wax, what should you do?

   _____

   _____

   _____

4. Why is pregnancy a contraindication for a hair removal treatment?

   _____

HIRSUTISM AND HYPERTRICHOSIS

1. What is the difference between hypertrichosis and hirsutism?

   Hypertrichosis: _____

   _____

   _____

   Hirsutism: _____

   _____

   _____

2. What are causes of hypertrichosis?

   • Congenital (acquired from birth)

   • _____ independent

   • Natural life occurrences, for example _____

- _____ to certain medical procedures
- Result of some _____ treatments
- Reaction to certain _____ , especially _____

3. What are causes of hirsutism?

- _____ inherited
- _____ dependent
- Diseases and disorders of the _____ system

4. What is the rare disorder of female clients with a beard called?

_____ Syndrome, and her "beard" is _____

THREADING

1. Fill in the blanks in the following questions with the words from the word bank.

banding	khite
faster rate	looped and twisted
fatlah	skin

a. Threading is also known as _____.

b. Threading is a method of hair removal that uses a _____ cotton thread maneuvered by the technician's fingers.

c. Threading does not cause trauma to the _____.

d. In Arabic, threading is known as _____ and, in Egyptian, _____.

e. Threading is mass tweezing but is accomplished at a much _____ then tweezing.

2. Explain the preparation of equipment and treatment area:

_____
_____
_____

3. Explain how you should prepare a client for a treatment:

_____
_____
_____
_____
_____

4. How long should the thread be? _____

SUGARING

Answer the following questions.

1. Where has sugaring been used for centuries? _____

_____

2. How long does the hair need to be? _____

3. What is the downside to sugaring? _____

4. What is the benefit to the spatula-applied method?_____

_____

5. Explain how the sugar paste should be applied to the skin:

_____

_____

_____

_____

_____

6. What are the benefits of sugaring?

a. _____

b. _____

_____

c. _____

_____

_____

d. _____

_____

_____

e. _____

f. _____

_____

_____

g. _____

_____

h. _____

i. _____
_____

j. _____
_____

k. _____

l. _____

m. _____

HARD WAX

Answer the following questions.

1. Why did hard wax make a comeback? _____
_____

2. What should the temperature be on the hard wax warmer?
_____

3. Depilatory waxes are often made up of beeswax, candelilla wax, and _____.

4. How should strip wax be applied?_____
_____
_____
_____

SOFT WAX

Answer the following questions.

1. Why is soft wax the most popular method?_____
_____
_____

2. What are some soothing ingredients found in soft wax?_____
_____

3. Why would a client experience small pustules a few days after a lip wax?
_____
_____
_____

4. What type of treatment would help ingrown hairs?_____

ADVANCED FACIAL WAXING

Answer the following questions.

1. On the illustration below, mark the direction you would measure for the beginning, arch, and end of the eyebrow.

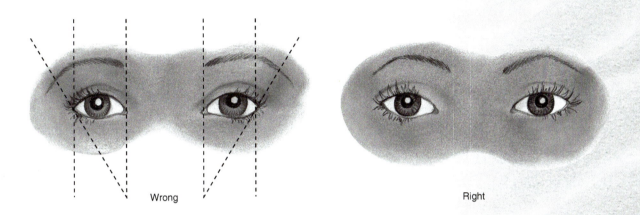

Wrong   Right

2. Draw the correct eyebrows on the face shape.

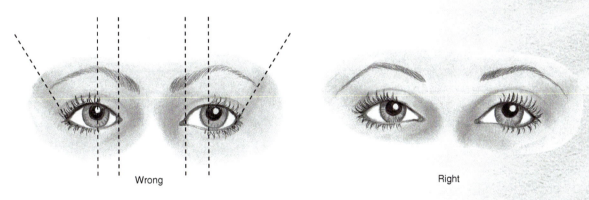

Wrong   Right

3. What type of wax is better for waxing the sides of the face and why?

_____

_____

SPEED WAXING AND BODY TECHNIQUES

Answer the following questions.

1. How is speed waxing accomplished?

_____

_____

2. In order to be an effective speed waxer, what should you do first?

_____

3. What is the most effective way to remove hair from the arms? _____

4. What is the most preferred method to wax the hands? _____

5. Describe the American bikini wax:

_____

_____

6. Describe a French bikini wax:

_____

_____

7. Describe a Brazilian bikini wax:

_____

THE BRAZILIAN WAX PROCEDURE

Fill in the missing steps for the Brazilian wax procedure

Procedure

1. Wash hands and put on gloves and an apron.

2. Fold back disposable drape and cleanse area with an antiseptic cleanser.

3. _____

_____

4. _____

5. Have the client sanitize hands if she will be helping to stretch the skin.

6. Test the wax.

7. _____

_____

8. _____

9. The femoral ridge is caused by a tendon on the inner thigh. This is an area that should not be waxed across in one pull.

10. _____

_____

11. DO NOT DOUBLE DIP! After each application, discard the disposable applicator in the trash.

12. Remove the soft wax in the normal manner.

13. _____

14. Apply second application of soft wax.

15. _____

16. Apply first application to side closest to you.

17. _____

18. Apply soft wax to hair at the top of the pubis, avoiding where the hairs converge.

19. Application of soft wax on the pubis.

20. Removal of soft wax to hair on the pubis.

21. _____

22. _____

23. Remove hard wax on pubis.

24. Apply pre-wax oil to labia furthest away from you.

25. Apply hard wax to labia furthest away from you in small strips with a smaller applicator.

26. Remove hard wax from labia,

27. _____

28. Remove hard wax on labia closest to you.

29. _____
_____

30. Apply soft wax downward with leg lifted.

31. Remove the wax upward removal with leg lifted.

32. Clients who have very little growth and the benefit of good mobility can assume the position shown.

33. Clients who have moderate to heavy growth and also poor mobility can assume the position in photo 38.

34. Clients who have moderate to heavy growth but good mobility can assume the position in photo 39.

35. _____

36. _____

37. Apply aftercare with a gauze square.

38. Give client post-care instructions

ADVANCED MALE WAXING

1. List the areas where men usually get waxed:

a. _____

b. _____

c. _____

d. _____

2. List the two areas that male swimmers get waxed:

a. _____

b. _____

3. When providing services to transgender clients, you may find these situations awkward. How would you handle these clients?_____
_____
_____

4. Describe an eyebrow wax for a man:

_____
_____
_____
_____
_____
_____.

5. In which direction should you wax a back? _____
_____

6. Explain how to wax a man's ears:

_____
_____
_____
_____
_____
_____

_____

_____

_____

_____

_____

ELECTROLYSIS

Fill in the blanks in the following questions with the words from the word bank.

laser	chlorine	ionization	positive
reduction	vellus	sodium hydroxide	hydrogen
permanent hair removal	FDA	diathermy	lye
producing heat	terminal	oscillating radio high-frequency waves	papilla
direct current	electrocoagulation	follicle	
chemical	negative	dermal papilla	

1. Electrolysis is currently the only proven method of _____
   recognized by the _____, though it does now recognize that _____ hair removal
   offers permanent _____. Unlike laser hair removal, electrolysis can be performed
   successfully on all types of hair: blond, dark, gray, straight, curly, _____, or
   _____.

2. Thermolysis, also called _____, is a method that uses _____ to produce
   _____. The high-frequency waves travel down
   the probe, and when the probe is placed in the _____ and surrounded by the
   moisture of the soft tissue cells, the water molecules of the soft tissue start to vibrate,
   _____. This heat causes tissue damage called _____ and
   can destroy the _____.

3. Galvanic modality uses _____, which flows in one direction, from
   the _____ pole to the _____ pole. The client holds an electrode (e.g., a
   handheld metal rod) carrying a positive charge of electricity, and the probe, which is
   negatively charged, is inserted into the _____. The result is that the current flows
   from negative to positive and an electrolytic _____ action, called _____,
   occurs to form one molecule of _____ gas, one molecule of _____ gas, and
   two molecules of _____ (NaOH), also known as _____. It is the _____
   that effectively decomposes the dermal _____.

COMPARATIVE FACTS FOR LASER HAIR REMOVAL VERSUS ELECTROLYSIS

Fill in the missing comparative facts for laser hair removal versus electrolysis.

Laser Hair Removal	Electrolysis
Permanent _____ , *not* _____ removal.[1]	_____ hair removal.
Not effective on hair lacking pigment, like gray or blond, or on vellus hair.	_____ _____
Not effective on _____ skin tones like Fitzpatrick _____.	Suitable for all skin tones.
Not a precise method, therefore not suitable for _____.	Selective, hair-by-hair method, perfect for _____ _____.
_____ _____	Perfect for finishing up the smaller percentage of regrowth hairs post laser.
Certain devices are more effective on hair and skin types than others.[2]	All electrolysis devices capable of three modalities: _____ _____; effectively treat all hair types.
_____ is required in most states.	No supervision is required.

HAIR REMOVAL AND PLASTIC SURGERY

Describe the stages that a male has to go through to complete the transgender reassignment to female.

1. Emotional and psychological counseling: _____
   _____
   _____
   _____

2. Hormone replacement therapy (HRT): _____
   _____
   _____
   _____
   _____

3. Reassignment surgeries: _____

_____

_____

_____

_____

_____

_____

_____

Date: _____

Rating: _____

MINERAL MAKEUP

Answer the following questions by using the words from the word bank.

70 percent to 90 percent	excellent	mica
1994	facial spritz	minerals
bismusth oxychloride	fine lines	slip and glide
boron nitrides	inert	sunscreen
breathe and function	iron oxide	weightless
chemical sunscreen	jawline	zinc oxide
dimethicone	kabuki	

1. When was the term coined to describe a concentrated pigment powder that was unlike the widely used, predominantly talc-based formulae found throughout the cosmetic world? _____

2. Traditionally, color cosmetics—base, blush and eye shadows—contain _____ _____ talcum powder.

3. Some of the mineral makeup usually contains a selection of the following minerals: titanium dioxide, zinc oxide, _____,bismuth oxychloride, boron nitride, and iron oxides.

4. Minerals used in powders are inert substances. _____ describes something that cannot support bacterial life.

5. Titanium dioxide is one of two ingredients approved by the FDA as a physical _____.

6. _____ is commonly used as a coating to increase the light-scattering properties of TiO_2.

7. _____ is also approved by the FDA as a physical sunscreen.

8. Mica gives _____ to the finished product.

9. _____ is a synthetically prepared, iridescent white or nearly white powder.

10. _____ is a white, silky powder that gives smoothness, coverage, slip, and sheen to the finished product.

11. _____, commonly known as rust, is primarily used as a colorant.

12. Mineral makeup gives _____ coverage with very little product.

13. When applied to clean, moisturized skin, these particles cling together and create a surface tension that overcomes gravity and hold the _____ tightly to the skin.

14. Minerals allow the skin to _____ normally.

15. A mineral makeup with an SPF can eliminate the need for _____ or enhance its protection.

16. If minerals are applied properly, they should feel _____ on the skin.

17. Foundation that is too dark will exaggerate _____ and accentuate pores.

18. To test the foundation color correctly, you should test it on the _____.

19. The best tool for loose mineral powder is a _____ or chisel powder brush.

20. If the minerals look powdery, wait a few minutes for the skin's natural oils to emerge or you may speed the process by using a _____.

APPLICATION PROBLEMS

List and explain three application problems.

1. _____
_____
_____
_____

2. _____
_____
_____

3. _____
_____
_____

APPLYING MINERAL MAKEUP

Find the following terms in the word search puzzle.

brushes   moisturizer

cleanser   tissues

drape   towel

gloves   sponges

mineral powders

```
J  U  P  W  B  L  X  Y  V  T  K  Z  K  A  X  G  K  O  J  L
C  V  X  T  I  S  S  U  E  S  H  H  V  F  E  I  I  J  A  P
Q  S  N  V  O  T  I  G  F  P  Y  F  K  S  A  Z  I  R  O  J
K  C  V  X  H  Z  V  J  Z  Z  T  E  E  Z  S  R  O  Y  O  W
S  S  E  O  R  N  P  W  M  H  Y  O  V  F  E  E  M  G  H  O
Q  U  E  J  G  V  E  E  S  D  Z  T  W  S  Q  H  O  D  V  F
B  X  U  J  X  Z  D  D  Q  K  Q  H  N  E  L  Y  I  X  U  B
O  L  Q  Y  Y  A  M  F  I  F  S  A  K  V  L  J  S  K  V  P
B  F  Y  S  E  G  N  O  P  S  E  L  U  C  X  T  T  P  P  I
X  M  Q  S  C  U  M  T  Y  L  D  Q  M  T  C  I  U  D  P  W
V  K  H  T  N  Z  Y  C  C  A  G  T  E  B  G  D  R  Q  A  A
S  Z  U  Y  S  R  E  D  W  O  P  L  A  R  E  N  I  M  L  P
Y  M  C  N  N  H  Q  Z  Y  T  U  T  N  W  V  E  Z  A  N  K
T  K  S  E  V  O  L  G  N  C  U  C  T  P  G  P  E  V  I  W
G  U  R  G  G  N  M  Q  L  O  A  N  O  I  F  H  R  L  D  N
O  K  V  K  Z  J  W  S  C  I  U  Q  T  V  E  N  O  Y  Z  I
Z  B  C  Q  F  U  F  B  A  P  X  J  V  P  F  J  T  S  S  O
I  B  S  E  H  S  U  R  B  C  Y  P  A  V  X  D  P  X  U  Q
Y  N  E  A  X  L  D  N  Y  R  P  R  Q  U  R  C  T  E  L  O
F  O  X  Z  O  B  R  E  R  U  D  Y  G  F  H  U  M  X  T  B
```

MINERALS FOR CAMOUFLAGE

Answer the following questions.

1. Even though green has been used for a long time in the makeup world to cover redness, _____ is all you need to neutralize red in the skin.

2. What are some of the reasons someone can get dark circles under the eyes?

a. _____

b. _____

c. _____

d. _____

e. _____

f. _____

g. _____

3. How should circles under the eyes be concealed?

_____

_____

4. What are two types of mineral under-eye concealer? _____

5. Cream mineral under-eye concealers usually come in a variety of _____ tones.

6. Yellow will be your best friend for covering the _____ in bruises and tattoos.

7. To conceal yellow bruising, using a _____ concealer can often be helpful. Simplify the process by using a _____ mineral powder.

AIRBRUSH MAKEUP

1. What are the two actions you can take using a dual-action airbrush?

_____

_____

2. What size airbrush nozzles should be used during the following procedures?

a. airbrushing beauty makeup _____

b. airbrushing body makeup _____

c. airbrush tanning _____

3. How do you accomplish a narrow spray pattern?

_____

_____

_____

_____

4. How do you accomplish a wide spray pattern?

_____

_____

_____

_____

5. How often should an airbrush be cleaned?

_____

_____

MAXIMUM COVERAGE AIRBRUSHING

Unscramble this list of materials and implements.

riarsubh teeqpimun   _____

irasuhbr daonufoinst   _____

dpsioalseb ogensp   _____

etstgni wdpreo   _____

repad   _____

dnehbada   _____

posisaldeb upc   _____

tsreifk   _____

levgos   _____

MAXIMUM COVERAGE AIRBRUSHING PROCEDURE

Write these procedure steps on a 3" × 5" card for reference.

Preparation

1. Prepare the work area for makeup application.

2. _____

3. Gather supplies.

4. Review the client's history to assure there are no breathing issues such as asthma which would make air brushing contraindicated before proceeding.

5. Review the client's expectations and the procedure.

Procedure

6. Seat and drape the client. Protect hair, if appropriate.

7. _____

8. If covering a tattoo, shave the area of all invisible hairs. Use colorless powder instead of shaving cream.

9. Use a water-based makeup, select a foundation color that matches the primary skin tone that surrounds the discoloration. Keep this color aside. You will use it for the final layer.

10. _____
    _____

11. Use the neutralizing color with a light touch targeting the natural shape of the hyperpigmentation or the design of the tattoo.

12. _____
    _____

13. _____

14. Repeat these two steps to achieve coverage.

15. When using alcohol-based makeup, it is not necessary to powder in between layers.

16. _____
    _____

17. When you have achieved 90 percent coverage and neutralization, rinse the airbrush to remove excess makeup:

18. _____
    _____

19. _____

20. If the skin's surface has freckles, you will need to reintroduce them.

21. Create a stencil with frisket film. It can be pierced with a pin to create odd-shaped holes, re-creating freckles. (For more details on frisket film, see the section later in this chapter on fantasy makeup.)

22. Using the freckle stencil, apply the freckle tone. Rotate the stencil and reapply. Repeat this process until the freckles match the surrounding area.

23. Finish with no-color setting powder.

24. When complete, rinse airbrush cup to clean the foundation from it.

SPRAY TANNING

1. Spray tanning should be applied in a single even layer and allowed to "_____" completely before applying another layer. Most manufacturers recommend waiting at least _____ before applying another coat of color.

2. The key ingredient in all spray tanning lotions is _____ or DHA. This is a colorless sugar derivative commonly obtained from sugar cane and sugar beets and from the fermentation of _____.

Write these key points on a 3" × 5" card for future reference.

SPRAY TAN CONCENTRATIONS (6–12 percent)

Very fair clients and a light tan _____

Fitzpatrick I–IV _____

Fitzpatrick > III dark tan _____

Stage competition _____

Pre- and Post-Treatment Education for the Client:

- Well _____ but no waxing just prior to visit.

- Oils or lotions may _____ of the tanning agent.

- Wear loose _____.

- Avoid getting the spray-tanned area wet for at least _____ hours.

- Use of many bar soaps may _____ the life of the tan.

- Avoid scrubbing or showering the area for at least _____ hours.

- The more frequently the client _____, the quicker the tan will fade.

- Routine use of lotions/oils will increase the duration of the tan once it has _____.

CONSIDERATIONS:

- Is there _____ and control of overspray?

- Are there any _____ issues?

- What is the developed color of the _____? Does it turn _____?

- What _____ are available? Do you know how to operate and maintain the equipment?

- What will be needed for _____ during the spraying process?

EYELASH PERMING

Answer the following questions.

1. What two other services can you offer for eyelashes?

a. _____

b. _____

2. What is the purpose of perming eyelashes? _____

_____

3. How long should you wait to apply eyelash extensions after perming the eyelashes? _____

4. How long should you wait to tint eyelashes after perming them? _____

EYELASH PERMING PROCEDURE

Find the following terms in the word search puzzle below.

applicator	hand mirror
clean towel	perming lotion
cotton swab	timer
glue	warm water

M	R	N	Y	F	E	T	L	R	J	R	R	T	F	D	A	Z	S	Y	B
V	Y	O	P	C	Z	N	B	U	P	D	K	M	P	R	W	Y	U	X	U
U	R	K	T	A	S	P	A	P	G	H	J	F	E	O	K	R	U	V	I
H	N	I	D	A	M	E	W	J	G	C	A	B	R	R	G	T	C	E	X
G	S	O	J	W	C	O	G	B	H	X	M	P	M	R	S	P	L	S	Z
V	B	T	M	E	T	I	J	T	D	I	R	I	I	I	W	Q	T	C	H
W	L	P	Q	V	U	X	L	I	Q	P	S	I	N	M	J	V	M	I	R
N	E	Y	C	O	P	L	K	P	P	D	A	V	G	D	W	Q	G	B	C
A	U	C	J	T	V	W	G	R	P	C	U	U	L	N	F	Z	A	M	L
G	J	C	L	Z	H	C	F	U	S	A	K	Z	O	A	E	W	U	R	H
J	T	E	T	E	L	L	F	K	A	F	E	W	T	H	S	E	D	H	T
A	E	W	H	O	A	Y	K	X	T	L	N	Y	I	N	G	Y	G	M	J
L	T	C	A	K	F	N	Z	W	T	I	J	Z	O	H	Q	Z	S	Z	D
O	J	R	L	R	H	Y	T	T	N	W	M	T	N	D	B	Z	J	P	V
M	L	H	D	S	M	L	Q	O	V	J	T	E	H	L	J	U	O	U	O
N	J	M	C	H	O	W	E	F	W	O	D	N	R	K	A	L	E	M	J
K	G	V	P	D	U	J	A	H	C	E	O	O	B	G	X	M	O	I	M
D	F	X	B	A	T	I	H	T	Y	C	L	C	K	L	L	A	X	A	F
R	A	E	X	G	M	A	F	H	E	D	Y	S	M	E	K	O	A	D	A
Z	K	O	C	W	P	W	F	S	U	R	V	I	K	E	C	Y	E	G	N

Fill in the missing steps in the following procedure and write this procedure on a 3" × 5" card for future reference.

1. Roller size guideline:

Smaller rollers: _____

Medium rollers: _____

Large rollers: _____

2. Cleanse the eyelashes, removing all eye makeup.

3. _____

4. The rollers are self-adhesive, so be careful to handle them only at the tips. Bend the roller slightly to fit the shape of the eyelid and trim the rod to the appropriate length of the eyelid.

5. Apply eyelash perming glue in a line at the base of the lashes and position the roller as close as possible to the root of the lashes. After positioning the roller, add more glue on the top of the roller.

6. _____

_____

_____

7. Apply perm solution with a cotton swab or manufacturer's applicator across the lashes adhered to the rod. Avoid contact with the skin. Carefully follow manufacturer's instructions; depending on the kit, timing ranges anywhere from 8 to 15 minutes.

8. _____

_____

_____

_____

9. Apply setting or neutralizer lotion to lashes with application stick. Leave neutralizer on according to manufacturer's instructions, generally 5 to 10 minutes.

10. _____

_____

11. If the kit includes a post-treatment lotion, apply it on an applicator stick or cotton swab. Let lotion set for five minutes or according to manufacturer's instruction.

12. _____

_____

_____

13. Clean lashes with a warm, damp cloth.

SEMI-PERMANENT EYELASH EXTENSIONS

Answer the following questions using the word bank below.

one-third	flush
catagen	four to six
closed	pregnancy
disinfection	protect
disposables	

1. Semipermanent lashes can last up to _____ weeks with the right combination of products, adhesive, and proper application.

2. Contraindications to lash extensions are _____, eye irritations, eye allergies, blepharitis, glaucoma, excessive tearing, and thyroid problems.

3. When applying lashes, you should follow all sterilization and _____ guidelines.

4. If adhesive should get in the eye, immediately _____ with plenty of water and contact a physician.

5. The client's eyes should remain _____ during the entire procedure, and at no time should adhesive be allowed to enter the eye.

6. The main purpose of the eyelash and eyelid is to _____ the eye from harmful substances or objects.

7. The three stages in a life cycle of a hair are anagen, _____, and telogen.

8. The use of as many _____ as possible will speed up your cleanup and minimize the sterilization process.

9. Three different types of looks can be accomplished by applying different lengths of lashes. For a natural look you would select lashes that are one-quarter longer than the client's lashes. For a feminine look, select lashes that are _____ longer than the client's lashes, and for a dramatic look, select lashes half again as long as the client's lashes.

10. Look for the following terms in the word search puzzle.

adhesive	lash comb
cotton swab	micro swab
disposable	tweezers
eye makeup remover	under-eye pad
headband	

```
W R K M Z E C O I K V F W H R L L N G J
K B M R R T L Y G L J G P I R B B N H S
X N A Z W S C C F I C I T W F C B L U B
I G R Z F B C O T T O N S W A B H M J D
Q U S B J U N R J T J P N M L Q G O U T
F F A D H E S I V E D K W I R I M V I U
Y F W E L W Z E Q N Z T F C O W M O W D
M D Q C L W Y Q O M T G O R T F Z D D E
P E Y E M A K E U P R E M O V E R I T U
D D I Y Q E Y H B T G W G S G G S S V E
R G L O P P M M Q S R L I W A F F P N X
U E N K I D O H F G W G I A M D O O Q J
L Y R Z G C Y P W H D L S B H L E S O P
K Z D F H O A P C C Z R J N H Z V A F P
R M E S D Z W T R K E N A G I C U B R I
Z N A W P B P K N Z Q H C F S P J L N M
G L L U N D E R E Y E P A D S U C E P B
O E I J W C T E Q O S E J E L J V Q P K
D P I S V H W J W A G N T R B D W Z N M
J A B G O T R J A C J H E A D B A N D C
```

TECHNIQUE VARIATIONS

Answer the following questions.

1. For a larger, more open-eye look you can:

a. _____

b. _____

c. _____

2. To create a thick, lush, glamour look:

a. _____

b. _____

HOME-CARE INSTRUCTIONS

List the post-application instructions for the client.

1. _____
_____

2. _____

3. _____
_____

4. _____

5. _____
_____

6. _____
_____

COMMON REASONS LASH EXTENSIONS FALL OFF

List the common reasons lash extensions fall off.

1. _____
_____

2. _____

3. _____

4. _____

5. _____

PERMANENT COSMETICS

Use the terms in the word bank to fill in answers for the questions.

advanced	medical condition
estheticians	rotary or digital rotary
eyeliner	single
hands-on	tattooing
aspirin, the use of topical	vigorous exercise, dirty or dusty environments, and swimming
one to five	UV, medications, lifestyle

1. The Society of Permanent Cosmetic Professionals (SPCP) Vision 2009 study results show that 31.5 percent of all permanent cosmetic technicians are also _____.

2. In 2006, the governor of Oklahoma signed a bill legalizing _____ and permanent cosmetics; they are now recognized and legal throughout the United States.

3. Those wanting to learn permanent cosmetics should recognize that it is a skill that can only be achieved with _____ training and lots of practice.

4. A fundamental training is in eyebrows, _____, and an introduction to lip-liner.

5. Full lip color is considered an _____ procedure, as are areola repigmentation, cheek color, eye shadow, or scar camouflage.

6. The common types of equipment include the manual method, _____, and coil.

7. If the client has a _____ that could affect the healing process, he or she would be directed to consult a physician and obtain a medical release before the procedure is performed.

8. Regardless of the equipment or device being used for the permanent makeup process, needles and pigments are considered _____ use.

9. Clients should be educated as to the process of the tattooing procedure, pre-procedure considerations such as avoiding _____ anesthetics, and care for their new permanent cosmetics.

10. _____ all must be avoided during the initial healing process to prevent the risk of infection and color loss.

11. All pigments fade, and re-enhancement may be needed in _____ years or longer depending on the exposure to _____, and many other factors.

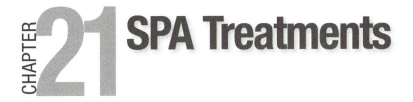

CHAPTER 21 SPA Treatments

Date: _____

Rating: _____

UNDERSTANDING SPAS AND THEIR SERVICES

Answer the following questions.

1. How many types of spas are there? _____ Describe each below.

2. Day spa: _____
_____
_____
_____

3. Destination spa: _____
_____
_____
_____
_____
_____
_____

4. Resort spa: _____
_____
_____
_____
_____

5. Medical spa: _____
_____
_____
_____
_____
_____
_____
_____
_____
_____
_____
_____

6. Fitness/health clubs: _____

_____

_____

_____

_____

_____

_____

_____

_____

7. Hospitals and rehabilitation facilities: _____

_____

_____

_____

8. Wellness centers: _____

_____

_____

_____

_____

_____

9. What types of tables are used for body treatments?

_____

10. Describe a wet table: _____

_____

_____

_____

11. What is the HIPAA law?

_____

12. What information do you need to obtain prior to giving a body treatment service?

_____

13. List the contradictions for a body treatment:

a. _____

b. _____

c. _____

d. _____

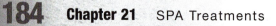

e. _____

f. _____

g. _____

h. _____

i. _____

j. _____

k. _____

l. _____

m. _____

n. _____

o. _____

p. _____

q. _____

14. List the steps for the table setup:

a. _____

b. _____

c. _____

d. _____
_____

e. _____
_____

f. _____
_____

g. _____

h. _____

15. What should you tell your client to make him or her more comfortable?

_____

16. List the client preparation procedures:

a. _____
_____
_____
_____

b. _____
_____
_____
_____
_____
_____

c. _____
_____
_____
_____
_____
_____

d. _____
_____

17. What are some steps that can ensure your client's comfort?

a. _____

b. _____

c. _____

d. _____

e. _____

f. _____

18. Fill in the missing words in the following paragraph using words from the word bank below.

foils	showers
injuries	tepid
plastic	treatment

Help clients off of the _____ table slowly to avoid _____, as they may be unsteady after lying down for an extended period of time. During some treatments, you may escort or help your client into the shower. Before a client _____, check the water (temperature), setting it to cool, then _____ to help slowly lower his or her body temperature. If your treatment involves the use of _____ or _____, remove these and re-drape the client so that they do not slip and fall from the materials.

19. How should a body product be removed with hot towels?

_____

_____

_____

_____

_____

_____

_____

_____

_____

_____

PROCEDURE FOR A BODY SCRUB WITH HYDRATING PACK/MASK

Fill in the missing steps for the body scrub and hydrating pack/mask procedure.

Preparation

1. Prepare the table with the materials you will need; remember that the outermost layer of material represents the first treatment.

2. _____

3. Prepare hot, wet towels and place them in the towel cabinet.

4. Review client health history to ensure that the client is still a candidate for this treatment.

5. _____

_____

6. _____

Procedure

7. Prepare the body with a cleansing gel or lotion, depending on the client's skin type.

   a. Use light effleurage movements over the entire body.

   b. _____

8. Spray appropriate toner with the Lucas or other spray applicator of your choice.

9. _____

   a. _____

   b. For enhanced exfoliation, use a handheld or machine-aided brush.

   c. _____
     _____
     _____
     _____
     _____

   d. If a granular scrub is used, rinse with large, wet sponges or hot, moist towels. Remember to maintain proper draping, exposing only the area being worked on.

10. As in step 2, apply appropriate toner with applicator of your choice.

11. _____
   _____
   _____
   _____ If working on the back of the body, take this time to do a scalp massage. If doing the front of the body, use this time to give the client a hand or foot massage or treatment.

   a. Allow the mask to process.

   a-1. Cover the client well.

   a-2. Use this time to give the client a massage.

12. _____
   _____

   a. _____

13. _____

14. Help the client turn over, maintaining the appropriate draping protocols. Repeat this entire process on the other side of the body.

Post-procedure

15. Help the client get up off the bed carefully.

16. _____

Cleanup and Disinfection

17. Follow cleanup and disinfection procedures in accordance with state guidelines.

18. _____

COMMON INGREDIENTS USED IN BODY TREATMENTS

Match the ingredients with their definitions.

alpha hydroxy acid   Used to boost collagen synthesis _____

beta hydroxy acid   Skin exfoliant _____

caffeine   Also called China clay _____

collagen   Moisturizer that has conditioning properties _____

green tea extract   Also known as "cyclic acid" _____

hyaluronic acid   Is added to topical creams for its moisturizing benefits _____

kaolin   Has the ability to kill bacteria _____

shea butter   Contains "catechins" _____

sulfur   A stimulant _____

vitamin C   An example would be salicylic acid _____

SEAWEED WRAPS

Answer the following questions.

1. What benefits does a cocoon wrap offer?

_____

_____

_____

2. What are the benefits of a seaweed wrap?

_____

3. During a seaweed wrap, how is the body exfoliated before the algae is applied?

_____

PROCEDURE FOR APPLYING AND REMOVING A SEAWEED WRAP

Fill in the missing steps in the following procedure.

Preparation

1. Prepare the treatment table with a protective covering (such as a sheet, plastic protector sheet, wool blanket, cellophane sheet, or space blanket and a top sheet or towel).

2. _____

_____

3. Review client health history to ensure that the client is still a candidate for this treatment.

4. _____

5. _____
_____
_____

6. Pre-treat the client by cleansing and toning the skin, one area at a time, prior to masking.

7. _____

Procedure

8. If the client is female, instruct her to cross her arms (to hold the modesty towel into place), and assist her into a seated position.

9. _____
_____

　　a. _____

10. _____

11. _____

12. Apply the mixture to the legs and buttocks starting with the nearest leg. This is accomplished by gently raising the knees and applying the mixture to the backs of the legs to the buttocks.

13. _____

14. Pull the plastic drape across the leg over the mud, and reposition the towel.

15. _____

16. _____

17. Next fold up the layers or blankets onto the client. Use a towel around the neck to prevent heat loss. Process for the desired time, which is usually 25 minutes.

18. _____
_____
_____

19. Starting with the nearest leg, remove all product from front of the leg. Raise the knee to allow complete removal of product from the back of the leg. Shift the plastic out of the way and re-cover client with a clean towel.

20. Repeat this process with the opposite leg. To remove the plastic out from under the client, shift it as far as possible to the left side and have the client elevate his or her hips slightly to assist you. Slide the plastic completely from under the client's lower body, ensure that all product has been removed, and re-cover the client.

21. _____

22. _____

23. Apply the lotion to the opposite leg.

24. _____
_____

25. Apply lotion to the client's chest and arms. The stomach is optional.

26. _____

27. Remove the last of the plastic.

28. _____
_____
_____

Post-procedure

29. _____

30. _____

Cleanup and Disinfection

31. Follow cleanup and disinfection procedures in accordance with state guidelines.

32. _____

HERBAL WRAPS

Answer the following questions.

1. What are the Ace® bandages soaked in?

_____

2. What benefits do the herbs offer?

_____
_____

3. What is the definition for diaphoretic?

_____

4. What is a hydrocollator?

_____

_____

5. What is a moist heat unit?

_____

PROCEDURE FOR A HERBAL BODY WRAP

Fill in the missing steps for the procedure for a body wrap.

Preparation

1. Prepare the moist heat unit following manufacturer's directions. The suggested temperature range is 150°F to 185°F (66°C to 85°C).

2. _____

_____

3. _____

_____

4. _____

_____

5. Set up the treatment room in standard spa treatment manner, from the treatment bed outward:

   a. First: water protective cover

   b. Wool blanket

   c. Metallic spa sheet

   d. Body pack film (optional)

   e. Large bath towel (for dry brushing step)

   f. Spa towel across the head of the lounge

6. Review client health history to ensure that the client is still a candidate for this treatment.

7. _____

_____

8. Some technicians offer the client warm herbal tea to raise core body temperature. Alternatively, a client can take a shower or sit in the sauna.

9. _____

_____

_____

Procedure

10. _____

_____

_____

11. Assist the client back up from the bed, keeping him or her draped in a large bath sheet if nude.

12. _____

_____

_____

_____

_____

13. Assist the client back onto the bed lying face up on the sheet.

14. Quickly wrap the linen sheet around the client's entire body. (You can also layer the sheet.)

15. _____

_____

_____

16. Wrap the thermal blanket over the herbal wrap sheet.

17. Wrap the insulating blanket over the thermal blanket.

18. Wrap the wool blanket over the thermal blanket.

19. _____

a. _____

b. _____

20. Apply a cool, folded washcloth to the client's forehead and across the eyes. For additional comfort, you can place a pillow under his or her head. If the client gets too warm, open the blanket around the neck.

21. Leave the client wrapped for 20 to 30 minutes. During this time, perform a scalp massage or play soothing music.

22. After the wrap has processed, remove the layers slowly, allowing the client to get acclimated to the cooler temperature of the room.

23. _____

24. _____

_____

25. As this is a detoxifying treatment, no lotions should be applied.

26. Allow the client to lie back down and rest, if desired.

Post-procedure

27. Offer the client water to rehydrate.

28. _____

_____

29. _____

Cleanup and Disinfection

30. _____

31. Disinfect any implements following state guidelines.

32. Clean and disinfect the moist heat unit following the manufacturer's directions.

HERBS USED IN WRAPS

Write the letter of each herb next to its beneficial quality.

A. Allspice   _____ Astringent properties

B. Burdock   _____ Soothing

C. Sage   _____ Increase blood circulation

D. Comfrey   _____ Astringent; toning; stimulating

E. Eucalyptus   _____ Muscle relaxant

F. Basil   _____ Increases circulation; detoxifying agent

G. Clove   _____ Stimulating

H. Rosemary   _____ Soothing

I. Lavender   _____ Effective with arthritis

J. Ginger   _____ Relieves bruises and inflammation

WRAPPING AGENTS

Answer the following questions.

1. What purpose does a cellophane body wrap serve?

_____

_____

2. What purpose does a blanket wrap serve?

_____

_____

3. What purpose does a Kneipp body wrap serve?

_____

_____

_____

SOOTHING LEG TREATMENT

Fill in the missing steps in the following procedure.

Preparation

1. Prepare the treatment table with bottom linens and blankets.

2. _____

_____

3. Place a small plastic covering on top of this towel.

4. _____

5. _____

_____

6. Review client health history to ensure that the client is still a candidate for this treatment.

7. Tell the client what to expect during the treatment.

8. _____

_____

Procedure

9. _____

_____

_____

10. On the moist skin, begin applying a mixture of mineral water, fango mud, and exfoliating granules.

    a. _____

       _____

    b. _____

11. Using the same steps as above, remove the product thoroughly with warm, moist towels that have been soaked in mineral water and warmed in the towel cabinet.

    a. _____

       _____

    b. _____

12. Repeat this process for the left leg. As you remove product from this leg, slide the plastic drape from under the client and remove. The client is now lying on the towel on top of the second sheet of plastic.

13. _____

     _____

14. _____

15. Slide towel out from beneath client's legs so he or she is against the plastic. Using a large brush or your hands, layer fango mud onto right leg front and back.

    a. _____

       _____

    b. _____

16. Repeat this process on the other leg.

17. Cover client's legs with blankets to keep them warm. Leave mud in place for 20 minutes.

18. _____

19. _____

20. Repeat for left leg. Allow client to rest.

21. Starting with the right leg, remove mud completely. Rinse well and wipe with a warm, wet towel. Cover the client with the towel when complete.

22. Repeat the removal procedure on the left leg.

23. _____

_____

24. Repeat on the left leg.

Optional: If your license permits, you may finish with a drainage massage or employ pressotherapy.

Post-procedure

25. Offer the client water to rehydrate her.

26. Inform her of any specific post-treatment instructions.

Cleanup and Disinfection

27. _____

28. Disinfect any implements following state guidelines.

HYDROTHERAPY AND OTHER SPECIALTY TREATMENTS

Answer the following questions.

1. What is the first step to beginning a shower treatment?

_____

2. What should the water temperature be?

_____

3. What is a scotch hose?

_____

_____

4. What should the temperature of the water be during a scotch hose treatment?

_____

5. What types of "baths" are available in some resort spas?

_____

6. What is the key benefit for the client in a Vichy shower? _____

_____

_____

7. Describe music therapy.

_____

8. List the benefits of music therapy:

a. _____
_____

b. _____
_____

c. _____
_____

d. _____
_____

e. _____
_____

f. _____
_____

g. _____
_____
_____

h. _____
_____

i. _____
_____
_____

j. _____
_____
_____

k. _____

l. _____

CHAPTER 22 Complementary Wellness Therapies

Date: _____

Rating: _____

THE HISTORY OF ALTERNATIVE MEDICINE

Use the terms in the word bank to fill out the questions below.

aura	Kirlian cameras
balance	man
chakra	medicine
compassion	nature
energy	vibration
interchangeable	

1. What we now call complementary and alternative medicine (CAM) was once the only _____ .

2. Famous physicist Albert Einstein recognized the separation between nature and _____ as creating a prison.

3. Einstein said that the only way to free ourselves from this prison was by "widening our circle of _____ to embrace all living creatures, the whole of nature and its beauty."

ENERGY BASICS

1. The spirit of man, _____, and the universe are one and the same.

2. If someone is out of balance, nature can fill the void and restore the _____.

3. Everything in nature, including you, is fueled by this _____. When you are full of energy, you are _____; when lacking energy, you become stressed and/or ill.

4. Spirit, energy body, subtle energy body, or essence are _____ terms describing the vital life force energy of all living things.

5. The inner face is the subtle energy body that we refer to as the _____ *system*.

6. _____, invented by Russian couple Semyon and Valentine Kirlian in the 1930s, are used to photograph the colors of the aura so that people without psychic vision are able to see the energy of the chakras made visible.

Definitions:

7. What is an aura: _____

_____

8. What is Leaky Aura Syndrome?

_____

_____

ENERGY MANAGEMENT

Answer the following questions.

1. Explain energy management:

_____

_____

2. What are some of the things that can throw off your balance energetically?

a. _____

b. _____

c. _____

d. _____

e. _____

f. _____

THE FOUR ENERGY BODIES

Answer the following questions.

1. What is the mental body?

_____

_____

2. What is the emotional body? _____

3. What is the spirit or subtle energy body?

_____

4. Fill in the missing information in the chart.

The Four Intelligences as They Relate to the Physical, Mental, Emotional and Spirit Bodies		
Physical Body	Sensory Intelligence	_____ _____ _____ _____
_____	Cognitive Intelligence	_____ _____ _____ _____ _____ _____ _____
Emotional Body	Feeling Intelligence	_____ _____ _____ _____ _____ _____ _____
_____ _____	Intuitive Intelligence	_____ _____ _____ _____

KEEPING THE ENERGY BODIES IN BALANCE

1. _____ is an effective way to bring balance to the _____ and _____ bodies. Essential oils from plants and flowers contain volatile oils that are considered to be the plant's _____ These components react with centers in the human brain, triggering a _____.

2. Herbs are plant materials that are taken internally rather than inhaled. You may choose from capsules, tablets, teas, and herbal elixirs, which are also called _____. They work more on the _____ because they are ingested through the digestive tract and are assimilated through the body.

3. Another method for reenergizing and re-balancing is _____ in a mini-meditation.

MINI-MEDITATION AND BREATHING EXERCISE

Answer the following questions.

1. What are the benefits of controlled breathing?

_____

2. When performing deep breathing, think of what you would like more of and breathe in that quality. What thoughts should you exhale?

a. Breathe in acceptance and breathe out _____.

b. Breathe in confidence and breathe out _____.

c. Breathe in gratitude and breathe out _____.

d. Breathe in abundance and breathe out _____.

e. Breathe in peacefulness and breathe out _____.

f. Breathe in love and breathe out _____.

g. Breathe in awareness and breathe out _____.

THE CHAKRA SYSTEM

Answer the following questions.

1. What does the word *chakra* originate from?

_____

2. What is each chakra associated with?

_____

_____

3. Use the words in the word bank to complete the paragraph below.

chakras	intuitive
create	life
heart	place

Conscious awareness is developed with _____ 4 through 7. Operating through the upper chakras, you have use of all of your intelligences—feeling, _____, sensory, and cognitive. You have connection to your _____, voice, vision, and intuitive insight to _____ your life rather than react to it. You receive information from a conscious source and have a clear vision of the big picture and how you fit into the picture, and you are able to speak clearly about your vision from the heart. When you come from this _____, you feel at peace and comfortable in your own skin and environment; you are able to feel a sense of purpose and passion for _____.

REIKI HANDS-ON HEALING

1. What is Reiki? _____

_____

2. What does *Rei* mean? _____

3. What does *Ki* mean? _____

4. Who developed Reiki? _____

5. List the benefits of Reiki:

a. _____

b. _____

c. _____

d. _____

_____

e. _____

f. _____

g. _____

h. _____

i. _____

j. _____

k. _____

6. Explain what type of healing each Reiki class offers:

First degree: _____

Second degree: _____

Third degree: _____

BACH FLOWER REMEDIES

Answer the following questions.

1. Who developed the Bach Flower Essences? _____

2. How many flower essences were developed first? _____

3. List the benefits of each Bach Flower Remedy:

a. White chestnut _____

b. Walnut _____

c. Larch _____

d. Rock water _____

e. Vervain _____

f. Holly _____

g. Rescue remedy essence and cream _____

POPULAR HEALING STONES

Answer the following questions.

1. What are healing stones?

_____

_____

2. What are the four different types of stones?

a. Warm stones are _____ .

b. Muted stones are _____ .

c. Cool stones are _____ .

d. Cleansing stones are _____ .

3. Each color has its own frequency or _____ .

4. If you add white to a color, it is a _____ .

5. If you add black to a color, it is a _____ .

6. Colors opposite each other on the color wheel are called _____ .

7. Placing a complementary color on a chakra will _____ .

8. What is the contraindication of a red stone? _____

9. List the steps to sanitize and clear your stones:

a. _____

_____

_____

b. _____

_____

_____

c. _____

_____

_____

_____

- _____

_____

- _____

_____

STONES AND CHAKRAS

List the stones for each chakra and explain what benefit each gives.

First chakra _____

_____

First chakra _____

_____

_____

Second chakra _____

_____

_____

Third chakra _____

_____

_____

Fourth chakra _____

_____

_____

Fouth chakra _____

_____

_____

Fifth chakra _____

_____

Fifth chakra _____

_____

_____

_____

Sixth chakra _____

_____

_____

_____

Fourth and seventh chakra _____

_____

_____

_____

Seventh chakra _____

_____

_____

AN ALTERNATIVE THERAPIES WORD SEARCH

Find the following terms in the word search puzzle below.

balance	gemstone
chakra	leaky aura
citrine	mental
color	Reiki
energy body	soul

```
I  X  W  G  X  A  Q  M  C  A  B  X  A  S  J  M  R  I  T  P
N  F  J  G  I  R  E  D  Q  P  V  Q  O  T  E  A  R  F  L  X
P  V  O  Z  M  N  T  X  Y  P  N  U  Q  N  F  E  T  A  M  A
S  T  M  P  F  O  O  A  R  N  L  J  T  G  S  B  S  E  F  Z
A  L  A  K  B  W  W  A  C  B  Q  A  J  Q  W  P  N  Y  R  V
Q  L  T  Y  P  V  Y  O  Q  C  L  W  E  W  R  O  P  X  I  G
B  R  M  I  T  Z  Z  S  L  Z  K  M  S  A  T  R  M  A  G  Q
M  E  Z  Z  W  U  Q  U  P  Y  S  B  Z  S  Q  V  R  H  X  Z
X  N  Z  C  T  R  E  I  K  I  Q  F  M  E  H  K  A  K  T  P
B  I  Q  H  F  J  C  G  P  W  C  E  H  D  A  I  Y  H  J  O
C  R  V  G  W  W  C  V  E  L  G  W  K  H  X  D  T  E  N  Z
W  T  J  R  B  Z  N  H  E  V  Z  N  C  P  O  C  R  R  V  X
L  I  W  O  F  R  N  F  T  G  O  Y  Y  B  M  U  B  C  Y  O
E  C  Y  L  K  S  L  P  P  Y  J  L  Y  J  Q  X  C  D  V  B
W  L  Y  O  M  P  W  F  C  K  F  G  V  D  M  W  S  L  J  D
S  S  M  C  P  K  M  Y  I  A  R  U  A  Y  K  A  E  L  E  P
J  K  L  L  J  U  K  R  Y  E  I  L  K  O  D  V  L  Q  X  W
L  A  S  O  G  K  E  O  N  C  I  I  N  P  R  Y  E  P  A  T
E  C  N  A  L  A  B  E  V  J  L  J  L  Q  U  N  S  A  U  X
V  G  U  V  B  Z  Q  V  Y  Z  A  A  P  U  J  V  L  Z  L  D
```

23 Ayurveda Theory and Treatments

Date: _____

Rating: _____

WHAT ARE AYURVEDIC TREATMENTS?

Answer the following questions.

1. What does Ayurveda refer to? _____

_____

_____

2. Use the terms in the word bank to complete the paragraphs below.

acupuncture	kinesiology
astrology	body therapies
aromatherapy	herbal supplementation
foot reflexology	sound therapy

Ayurveda is the source of many types of _____ used today, including: _____, polarity therapy, full-body oil massage, deep tissue massage, _____, physiotherapy, _____, and hydrotherapy. It also gave birth to modern medical treatment approaches such as nutrition, _____, homeopathy, _____, psychiatry, and surgery, including cosmetic surgery.

Ayurveda provides insight from a wide variety of sources, including more esoteric studies such as _____; mantra or healing through prayer and chanting; color therapy; music or _____; gem therapy and the use of stones; and alchemical preparations.

3. Explain the five Vedic principles:

a. Sound: _____

_____

b. Sight: _____

_____

_____

c. Smell: _____

_____

_____

d. Touch: _____

_____

_____

e. Taste: _____

_____

_____

_____

f. Heart feeling: _____

_____

_____

4. What is the combination of subtle energies or five great elements called?

_____

THE THREE DOSHAS

1. Describe the three doshas:

a. Vata: _____

_____

_____

_____

_____

_____

_____

b. Pitta: _____

_____

_____

_____

_____

_____

_____

_____

c. Kapha: _____

_____

_____

_____

_____

_____

2. What does Prakuti mean? _____

3. What does Vikruti mean? _____

THE QUALITIES OF THE FIVE ELEMENTS

1. Explain the qualities of the five elements:

Space: _____

_____

Air: _____

_____

Fire: _____

_____

Water: _____

_____

Earth: _____

_____

2. If one element is allowed to accumulate, then problems will eventually manifest. What problems happen if there is:

Extra earth: _____

Extra water: _____

Extra fire: _____

Extra air: _____

Extra space: _____

VATA BODY–MIND CHARACTERISTICS

Answer the following questions.

1. The Vata body will appear as _____.

2. The Vata actions will be _____.

3. The Vata will talk about _____.

4. What unbalances the Vata dosha? _____

_____

_____

_____

_____

5. What can be done to balance the Vata dosha? _____

_____

_____

6. What are the key words to help customize a treatment for a Vata dosha?

_____

7. What treatment components would be the best for the Vata dosha? _____

_____

_____

_____

PITTA BODY–MIND CHARACTERISTICS

Answer the following questions.

1. The Pitta body will appear as _____

_____.

2. The Pitta movements will be _____.

3. The Pitta's speech will be _____.

4. What unbalances the Pitta dosha? _____

_____

_____

5. What can be done to balance the Pitta dosha? _____

_____

6. What are the key words to help customize a treatment for a Pitta dosha?

_____

7. What treatments or components would be best for the Pitta dosha? _____

_____

_____

_____

KAPHA BODY–MIND CHARACTERISTICS

Answer the following questions.

1. The Kapha body will appear as _____
_____.

2. The Kapha movements will be _____.

3. The Kapha's speech will be _____.

4. What unbalances the Kapha dosha? _____
_____
_____

5. What can be done to balance the Kapha dosha? _____
_____

6. What are the key words to help customize a treatment for a Kapha dosha?
_____

7. What treatments would be best for the Kapha dosha? _____
_____

CUSTOMIZED ESSENTIAL OIL BLENDS AND HERBS

Describe the oil blends and herbs for each dosha.

1. Vata blend: _____
_____
_____
_____
_____

2. Pitta blend: _____
_____
_____
_____
_____
_____

3. Kapha blend: _____
_____
_____
_____
_____

MAGICAL MARMAS

Answer the following questions.

1. What is a marma point? _____

2. How many marma points are there? _____

3. How does a marma point close? _____

BASIC MARMA POINT MASSAGE

Fill in the missing steps in the procedure below.

Preparation

1. _____

2. Gather supplies and products.

3. Warm the oil in a massage oil heater or other warming device.

4. Review the client's history with him or her and ensure the appropriateness of the procedure. Then select the appropriate Ayurvedic massage blend based on the client's dosha.

Procedure

5. _____
_____

6. Position 2, on the midline of the head, eight finger widths above the eyebrows. Using your thumb, middle finger, or fourth finger, perform 15 to 30 gentle clockwise circles.

7. _____
_____
_____
_____

8. _____
_____
_____

9. Position 5, place hands on both sides of the head at the top of the spine. Support the head with one hand and massage with the other, rotating your hands as needed to completely massage both sides of the head. Work deeply enough to manipulate the skin and muscles of the scalp. Use all of your finger tips to generally move over the scalp using sufficient pressure to gently move the scalp over the skull and systematically working over entire scalp.

10. _____

_____

_____

11. _____

_____

_____

12. _____

_____

13. _____

_____

_____

_____

14. Decant appropriate ayurvedic oil into palms of your hands but do not rub hands together.

15. _____

_____

16. _____

_____

_____

_____

17. Position 12, _____

_____

_____

18. _____ mid chin to temple, release using two fingers from each hand simultaneously.

19. Perform three press-release patterns on the center of the mentalis.

20. _____

_____

21. _____

_____

22. Position 16, _____

_____

_____

23. Position 17, _____

_____

24. _____

_____

25. _____

_____

26. _____

_____

27. Position 20, _____

_____

28. Position 21, perform five circles over right and left mastoid process.

29. _____ nostrils to mastoid. This is done one side of the face at a time. The hand not being used for massage is resting on the top of the client's head.

30. At the flare of the right nostril, where the nostril joins the face, perform three press-release patterns.

31. _____

_____

32. Position 24, chin to temple glide. Using two fingers of each hand, trace along the jawline from the center of the chin to the temple, and perform five circles on the temporal region.

33. _____ mid-nose to mastoid. This is performed on both sides of the face simultaneously. Starting at the point about halfway up either side of the nose at the level of the zygoma, perform three press-release patterns.

34. Position 26, slide across cheek bones toward the top of the ears then up and over behind the ears to the mastoid process.

35. Position 27, perform five circles on the mastoid process.

36. Position 28, under eyes. Perform one eye at a time with the other hand resting on the client's head for stability and security. All pressure in this area should be on the lower ridge of the orbital bone toward the toes of the client, not into the eye socket area.

   a. Starting at the inner corner of the eye socket, perform three press-release patterns.

   b. Glide about a quarter of the way toward the outer corner of the eye, and repeat three press-release patterns firmly enough to feel the boney eye socket under your thumb.

c. Glide about half of the way toward the outer corner of eye, and repeat same pattern.

d. Glide about three-quarters of the way toward the outer corner of the eye, and repeat three times pressing and releasing.

e. Again, glide to outer corner of the eye, and vibrate with your index finger using gentle pressure against the inner surface of the boney orbit of the eye socket.

37. _____

_____

   a. _____

_____

   b. _____

_____

   c. _____

   d. _____

   e. _____

   f. _____

   g. _____

38. _____

_____

a. Starting at the inner corners of the brow, gently but firmly pinch and release.

b. Shift one finger width toward the outer brow and repeat.

c. Repeat this pattern across the brow, ending at the outer corners.

39. Position 31, tip of nose-forehead spiral _____

_____

_____

40. Position 32, starting with a tiny circle and slowly enlarging, trace a spiral that grows to encompass the entire forehead.

41. Position 33, zigzags. This movement should be gradually quicker and a bit stimulating to slowly rouse the client.

   a. _____

_____

b. _____

_____

42. _____

_____

43. Position 35, now rest the thumbs very gently on the closed eyelids of the client and close the ears with the middle fingers. Hold for a minute and silently extend the wish that the treatment has been of benefit.

44. Remove any excess massage oil with a warm moist towel, wet disposable sponges, or cotton pads.

45. Complete with appropriate SPF product or move into additional facial steps as desired.

SHIRODHARA TREATMENT

Answer the following questions.

1. Explain the Shirodhara treatment: _____

_____

2. List the contraindications to the Shirodhara treatment:

a. _____

b. _____

c. _____

d. _____

e. _____

f. _____

g. _____

h. _____

i. _____

j. _____

CHAPTER 24

Working in a Medical Setting

Date: _____

Rating: _____

INTRODUCTION

Find the following terms in the word search puzzle below.

anecdotal	control group	medical spa	plastic surgeon
board certified	cosmetic dermatology	placebo	scope of practice

```
I D B P N Y Y X Q Q C A I O H N W G D W J X
C E I Y H F U M C R G C N G O U M M R Z Y F
O T U N I Z M V U O J N E E Q O P B T O J H
S W D T R D U I F W N E G E C Z M C B M U H
M E P J Y K E S D P R R C S D D Z C E G K Y
E S M V P S F P L V U B A P Z F O I Q Y B A
T B C Z A D S C L S J P K Y I R B T A B C O
I O P O A H B M C A S S U E G H O Y A K C W
C E Z F P P A I D L C M R M I A A H T L O Q
D X C A V E T H A A M E K T Z E R Y M N N Z
E A B W I S O C A M P J B Q U A D Q N L T W
R G J N A C I F G P S B O O K F C D W M R P
M C I L P D U V P B U D F B N P E Y Q G O B
A B P R E T N T S R Z Z O N S E R Q V J L Y
T F N M Y I N N J O A B W D J V T E W F G J
O Q P A M O I X I O G C V O C R I H Q V R I
L E X E X I H C S K I S T M W Z F X I G O N
O V O P U L F L U C A Q Z I T K I Y I T U Y
G G H K A T A I M D C Q K K C R E M Z Q P L
Y U B U Z A D Z R U S O O J J E D K J C M T
U E M X F R E M W Q E T U N E V F C Q N N B
F Q N E I O D N F L G H M F T P Y B D J L L
```

SCOPE OF PRACTICE

Answer the following questions.

1. What are some of the noninvasive procedures done in a medical spa?

   _____

2. When working in the medical field, you should always check with your state legislature for _____.

3. What are the educational requirements in your state? _____

   _____

4. What are the various types of doctors that an esthetician can work with?

   a. _____

   b. _____

   c. _____

   d. _____

   e. _____

5. What is the difference between a cosmetic surgeon and a reconstructive surgeon?

   _____

   _____

   _____

   _____

   _____

6. What kind of medical practices can "medical esthetics" be associated with? _____

   _____

7. What are two types of nurses? _____

   _____

8. It is imperative that we as estheticians working in a medical setting obtain _____ even if our respective states do not require further training.

9. Estheticians are familiar with working in accordance with _____ _____ standards in spas and salons; in a medical facility, observing the _____ rules and regulations are paramount.

THE SCIENTIFIC METHOD

Answer the following questions.

1. All medical protocols are based on the _____ a philosophy of reasoning that is based on first generating and then testing a _____.

2. Explain what the term "control group" means. _____
_____

3. What is a placebo? _____
_____

4. Name the five steps of the scientific method:

   a. _____

   b. _____

   c. _____

   d. _____

   e. _____

5. What is anecdotal evidence? _____
_____

6. What does the acronym SOAP stand for? _____

7. How do you refer to the patrons of a medical spa? _____

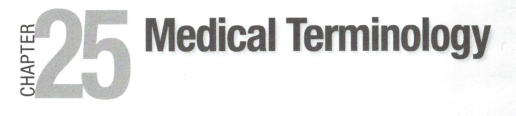

CHAPTER 25 Medical Terminology

Date: 2/18/2022

Rating: _____

HOW MEDICAL TERMINOLOGY WORKS

1. By knowing the meaning of a Greek or Latin _root words_, you can understand the meaning of an entire word. The use of _suffixes_ and _prefixes_ give further clarity.

2. What does the suffix *-ology* mean? ___the study of something___

3. What does the suffix *-graphy* mean? ___to record___

4. To find the suffix of a word, isolate the different parts of the word. Look for the _O_ _in the middle of the word_ or another _combining vowel_.

WORD ANALYSIS

Write the root part of the word next to the word itself.

opthalmoscope	ophthalm
polyneuropathy	neur
pathology	path
intravenous	ven
leukocyte	leuk
amniocentesis	amni

PLURALS

List the 10 common exceptions to basic plural rules.

1. ___-is___

2. ___-us___

3. ___-ix___

4. -ion _____

_____

5. vas _____

6. pons _____

7. ora _____

_____

8. femur _____

9. corna _____

10. panes _____

ROOT WORDS

Write the meaning next to each root.

1. adip   fat

2. andr   male

3. anth   flower

4. arc   arched

5. blephr   eyelid

6. bull   blister

7. carcin   cancer

8. call   hardened skin

9. capill   hair

10. cau   to burn

11. cheil; chil   lip

12. chir   hand

13. chrom; chromat-   color

14. coll(a)   glue

15. corn   horny

16. crine   secretion

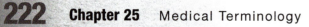

17. cut   skin

18. cyst   bladder

19. derm; dermlat   skin

20. ede   to swell

21. erythr   red

22. fibr   fiber

23. foll   bag

24. glab(r)   smooth

25. hem; hemet   blood

26. hepat, hepar   liver

27. hist; histi   tissue

28. ker; kerat   horny tissue

29. lacrim   tear

30. later   side

31. lept   delicate

32. lip   fat

33. lum   light

34. lymph   lymph

35. macul   spot

36. mal   cheek

37. melan   dark

38. morph   to form

39. nar   nostril

40. necr   dead tissue

41. nerv   nerve

42. neur   nerve

43. ocul   eye

44. op; opt _____ eye _____

45. opthalm _____ eye _____

46. ot _____ ear _____

47. path _____ disease _____

48. pell _____ skin _____

49. pil _____ hair _____

50. phleb _____ vein _____

51. phot _____ light _____

52. plas(t) _____ to form or mold _____

53. rhin; rhine _____ nose _____

54. sarc _____ flesh _____

55. scler _____ hardened _____

56. therm _____ heat _____

57. tox _____ poison _____

58. trich _____ hair _____

59. troph _____ development _____

PREFIXES

Write the meaning next to each prefix.

1. a, ab, abs _____ from _____

2. ad, ac, ag, al _____ near, to, toward _____

3. anti _____ opposite _____

4. circum _____ around _____

5. com; con; co _____ with _____

6. dys _____ bad, difficult _____

7. endo; ento _____ within _____

8. epi _____ upon _____

9. hyper _____ more _____

10. hypo _____ less _____

11. im; in _____ into, lack of _____

12. intra; intro _____ within _____

13. per _____ through, wrongly _____

14. peri _____ around, nearby _____

15. pro _____ before _____

16. pre _____ before _____

17. post _____ after, behind _____

18. pro _____ ~~to~~ forward, in front _____

19. re; red _____ again _____

20. retro _____ backward, back _____

21. se _____ away _____

22. sub; suc; suf; sup _____ under, somewhat _____

23. super; supra _____ above _____

24. sym _____ with, together _____

25. trans; tran; tra _____ across _____

26. ultra _____ beyond _____

SUFFIXES

Write the meaning next to each suffix.

1. -iac _____ a person afflicted with a disease _____

2. -ia _____ an unhealthy state _____

3. -is _____ forms the noun from the root _____

4. -ism _____ condition, state of being _____

5. -logy _____ study of _____

6. -gen _____ producer _____

7. -y _____ ~~forming or fixing~~ condition, process _____

8. -plasty _____ forming or fixing _____

9. -itis   inflammation

10. -icle

11. -al   relating to

12. -ate   status

13. -ectomy   surgical removal of a specified part of body

14. -emia   substance is present in the blood

15. -iasis   names of diseases

16. -in; -ine   belonging to

17. -ize   make or become

18. -phobia   irrational fear or dislike

19. -plasty   formation of a specified part of the body

20. -stomy   cutting a specified part of the body

21. -therapy   treatment intended to relieve ## or heal

22. -tomy   cutting a specified part of the body

23. -ency   denoting a quality

24. -itious   corresponding to nouns ending

PRONUNCIATION

How are the following letter combinations pronounced?

1. ph   f

2. ps   s

3. ch   k

4. mn   n

5. pt   t

6. pn   n

7. dys   dis

8. gn   n

9. x   z

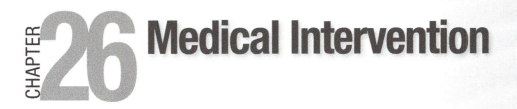

CHAPTER 26 Medical Intervention

Date: _____

Rating: _____

MEDICAL INTERVENTION DEFINED

Answer the following questions.

1. Give one example of non-surgical aesthetics. _____

2. What are the two sides of medical esthetics? _____

3. With what does the esthetic side primarily deal? _____
_____

4. About what type of medical procedures would an esthetician consult with a client?
_____
_____

5. What information should an esthetician discuss in regard to dermal fillers? _____
_____
_____

6. With what should the esthetician be intimately familiar? _____
_____

7. What is meant by the "durability" of products? _____
_____
_____

8. How do you choose the most durable product? _____
_____

AN INTRODUCTION TO BOTOX COMETICS/DYSPORT

Answer the following questions.

1. What are some of the complications with Botox Cosmetic? _____
_____
_____

2. In what areas would Botox Cosmetic be injected for wrinkles? _____
_____
_____

3. How long does Botox Cosmetic last? _____
_____

4. What is eyelid ptosis? _____
_____

5. Up until recently, what conditions has Botox been able to treat? _____
_____
_____

6. Botox Cosmetic is the product name for _____

7. List the indications for neurotoxins:

a. _____
_____

b. _____

c. _____

d. _____

e. _____

8. Use the words in the word bank to complete the following paragraph.

brow laxity	glabellar
droopiness	inexperienced
forehead	ptosis

Forehead lines are the horizontal lines that are created when the brow is lifted. Treating the _____ can be one of the more challenging indications because the depth of the lines may be an indication for potential _____. Complete relaxation can be responsible for brow _____, especially in the hands of the _____ injector professional. When discussing neurotoxin therapy for the brow with a client, the physician or nurse will look for several key indicators: brow heaviness or _____, lid heaviness, _____ involvement, and depth of lines.

9. Where are "crow's feet" ? _____

10. Where are "marionette lines"? _____
_____

11. What is another name for vertical lip lines? _____

12. What are the more serious yet uncommon adverse reactions associated with the use of Botox Cosmetic in the treatment of cervical dystonia and blepharoplasm?

    a. _____

    b. _____

    c. _____

    d. _____

13. What are complications and side effects of Dysport when treating cervical dystonia?

    a. _____

    b. _____

    c. _____

    d. _____

    e. _____

    f. _____

    g. _____

    h. _____

AN INTRODUCTION TO DERMAL FILLERS

Answer the following questions.

1. What are the positive qualities to a perfect injectable material?

    a. _____

    b. _____

2. What are the possible drawbacks of an injectable filler?

    a. _____

    b. _____

    c. _____

d. _____

e. _____

3. When it comes to injectable fillers, what is important to the client?

a. _____

b. _____

c. _____

d. _____

e. _____

f. _____

g. _____

4. Dermal fillers made of natural products include:

a. _____

b. _____

c. _____

5. Fill in the missing words within this paragraph using the word bank below.

extracellular	perfect
hyaluronic acid	polysaccharide
hypoallergenic	structure-stabilizing
natural volume	

Although other injectables are available _____ seems to hold the best hope for a _____ dermal filler. Meeting many of the criteria noted by professionals, such as durability. It is a _____ found in human tissue, as such _____ is _____. "Hyaluronic acid exists in the _____ space and functions as a space-filling, _____, and cell-protective molecule." In other words, hyaluronic acid is, in part, responsible for the _____ found in youthful skin, a perfect solution for dermal filling, it would seem.

6. Label the photographs as to what the indication is and what treatment would be the best.

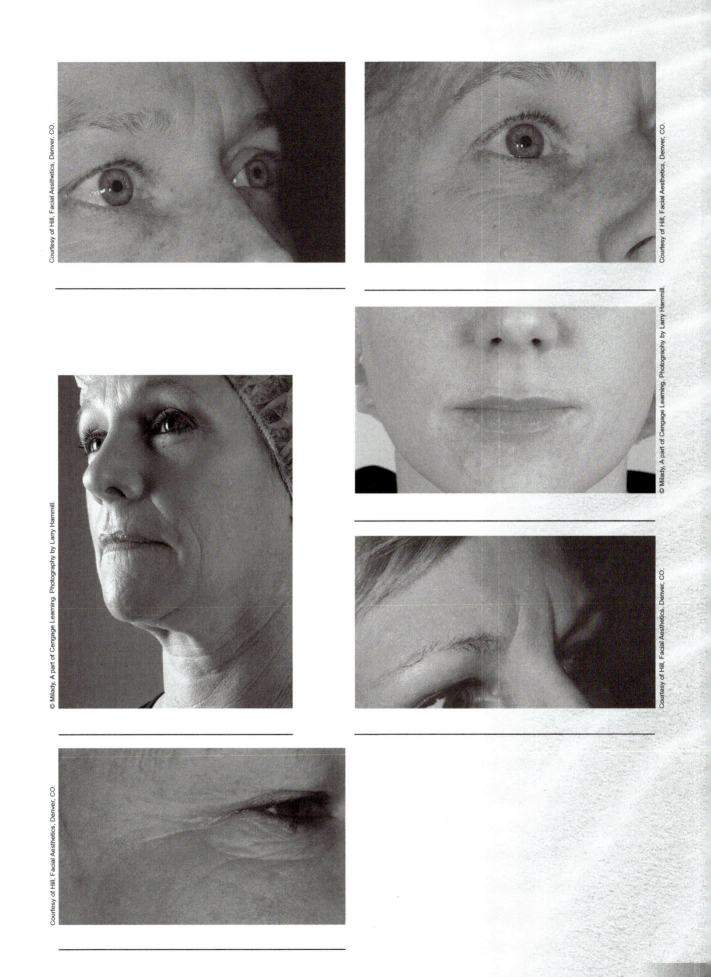

7. List synonyms for dermal filling

a. _____

b. _____

c. _____

d. _____

e. _____

8. List indications for dermal filling

a. _____

b. _____

c. _____

d. _____

e. _____

f. _____

g. _____

h. _____

i. _____

9. Why is hyaluronic acid the best hope for a perfect dermal filler?

_____

_____

_____

_____

10. Fill in the blanks.

a. Hyaluronic acid is a naturally occurring _____ sugar.

b. Fifty percent of the hyaluronic acid is housed in the _____.

c. Hyaluronic acid's chemical makeup enables it to hold up to _____ in weight in water.

d. The FDA-approved fillers with hyaluronic acid are _____, _____, _____, _____, _____.

e. The non-FDA-approved fillers with hyaluronic acid are _____
_____

11. Fill in the missing information in this chart.

Name of Product	FDA Approval	Manufacturer
Restylane®	_____	Q-Med
Restylane FINE LINE™© _____	_____	_____
*Restylane*PERLANE™© _____	Yes	_____
Juvederm®	_____	Allergan Promery Zone Artisanale de Pre Mairy, LEA Derm)
Juvederm Ultra®	_____	Allergan Promery Zone Artisanale de Pre Mairy
Macrolane®©	_____	_____
Prevelle®	_____	Mentor
Dermalive®©	_____	_____
DermaDeep®©	_____	Dermatech
Matridur®©	No	Medical Aesthetic Supplies
Matridex®©	_____	Medical Aesthetic Supplies
Viscontour®	No	Aventis Dermatology

12. When was Restylane FDA approved? _____

13. What are Restylane and Perlane synthesized from cultures of? _____
_____

14. What does NASHA stand for? _____

15. What treatments are Restylane and Perlane popular for? _____
_____

16. What is a common mistake when using dermal fillers in the lips? _____
_____

17. What are Juvederm and Juvederm Ultra Plus injectables intended for?
_____

18. What are Restylane, Perlane, Juvederm, and Juvederm Ultra Plus excellent choices for?

_____

_____

19. Fill in the blanks:

Prevelle Silk has a specific _____ to assist with durability. Prevelle is typically used for _____ such as the _____ or the _____ after Botox Cosmetic or Dysport. It is a short-acting hyaluronic acid filler and typically will not last as long as the more robust fillers such as _____ and _____ But every face is different and each skin type requires _____ ; the _____ of these products helps the injector to have a _____ available for client treatment.

20. Name two non-hyaluronic acid injectables and the intended treatment.

_____

_____

21. Describe how SCULPTRA® is administered:

_____

_____

_____

22. Fill in the blanks:

Radiesse© is _____ suspended in gel. The gel is made from _____. These components are _____, and the calcium hydroxylapatite is _____. Calcium hydroxylapatite has been used with _____ _____; it also is used for _____ because it has a _____ nature. Radiesse© is FDA approved for use in the _____ _____as well as for cosmetic uses.

23. What are examples of dermal filler complications?

_____

_____

_____

24. Fill in the blanks:

The dermal filler will hold for approximately _____ to _____ months (depending on the product used); the neurotoxin therapy will hold for _____ to _____ months.

INTRODUCTION TO SCLEROTHERAPY

Answer the following questions.

1. Use the words in the word bank to complete the paragraph below.

red, blue, or purple veins	valves
spider veins	varicose veins

Dilated blood vessels, also known as _____, are a problem for many people. They appear as _____ through the skin's surface, most often on the lower extremities. As we age, these can also be found on the hands, on the cheeks, and around the nose. These are a result of the failure of _____ within the veins. Most often varicose veins—and especially _____—are relatively harmless, even if they are unsightly.

2. Explain the three generalities of varicose veins:

a. Gender: _____
_____
_____

b. Geography: _____
_____
_____

c. Age: _____
_____
_____

3. How can the esthetician be helpful during sclerotherapy? _____
_____

4. What conditions would disqualify someone from having a sclerotherapy treatment?

a. _____

b. _____

c. _____

d. _____

e. _____

f. _____

g. _____

5. Explain the client preparation for sclerotherapy: _____

_____

INTRODUCTION TO MEDICAL PEELS

Answer the following questions.

1. Explain what a chemical peel does: _____

_____

2. What are the four levels of peeling?

    a. _____

    b. _____

    c. _____

    d. _____

3. What will chemical peeling help with? _____

4. List different types of peeling agents:

    a. _____

    b. _____

    c. _____

    d. _____

    e. _____

5. Glycolic comes from what plant? _____

6. In what strengths is glycolic available? _____

7. What does a Jessner's peel have in it? _____

_____

8. What type of peel is a Jessner's peel? _____

9. From what does salicylic acid derive? _____

10. In what strengths is a salicylic acid peel available? _____

11. If someone has a salicylate toxicity, what would the symptoms be? _____

_____

12. In what strengths is a TCA peel available? _____
_____

13. What is the most commonly recognized TCA peel? _____

14. How far deep into the skin does a TCA peel penetrate? _____
_____

OTHER SOLUTIONS

1. Fill in the missing information in the chart.

Treatment	These Treatments:	These Treatments Do Not:
Trichloracetic acid peels	Flatten scarring	_____
	Reduce rhytides	_____
	_____	_____
	Improve hyperpigmentation	_____
Jessner's solution and AHA and BHA acid peels	Reduce rhytides _____ _____	Reduce pore size _____ Remove telangiectases Remove deep scarring

2. What are the contraindications for chemical peeling? _____
_____

CHAPTER 27 Plastic Surgery Procedures

Date: _____

Rating: _____

FACE-LIFT (RHYTIDECTOMY)

Answer the following questions.

1. What is a rhytidectomy? _____

2. With what procedures is the rhytidectomy usually partnered? _____
_____

3. Along with the rhytidectomy, what skin resurfacing procedures can be used to fine-tune the facial skin? _____

4. What will a rhytidectomy treat? _____
_____
_____
_____

5. How many types of face-lift techniques are there? _____
_____

6. Why do people that smoke need to quit smoking one to two weeks before the surgery?
_____
_____

7. Explain the thread lift: _____
_____
_____
_____
_____

8. What does the thread lift treat? _____
_____

9. How long does this procedure take? _____

FOREHEAD-LIFT (BROW-LIFT)

Answer the following questions.

1. What does a forehead-lift treat? _____

2. What other surgeries might be performed at the same time to complement the forehead-lift? _____

3. What are the two main surgical techniques for the forehead-lift? _____
_____

4. How is the first technique performed? _____
_____

5. How is the second technique performed? _____
_____
_____

6. Where is the incision in the classic forehead-lift? _____
_____
_____

EYE-LIFT (BLEPHAROPLASTY)

Answer the following questions.

1. What is a blepharoplasty? _____

2. How many were performed in 2010? _____

3. What would a blepharoplasty treat? _____

4. What symptoms are not treated by a blepharoplasty? _____
_____

5. What information is obtained prior to a blepharoplasty? _____
_____

6. Which medical conditions would make the surgery risky? _____
_____

7. Describe the incision process in the case of altering the upper eyelids: _____
_____
_____

8. Describe the incision process in the case of altering the lower eyelids: _____
_____
_____
_____

9. What is a transconjunctival blepharoplasty? _____
_____

10. What is photophobia and when might it occur? _____
_____

NOSE JOB (RHINOPLASTY)

Answer the following questions.

1. What is a rhinoplasty? _____

2. Give an example of reconstructive rhinoplasty: _____
_____

3. What can contribute to nasal airway obstruction? _____
_____

4. Give an example of cosmetic rhinoplasty: _____
_____

5. What other surgeries can be performed with rhinoplasty? _____

6. Describe a rhinoplasty procedure: _____
_____
_____
_____

7. What can influence the outcome of the surgery? _____
_____
_____
_____

8. What are the two types of rhinoplasty? _____

FACIAL IMPLANTS

Answer the following questions.

1. What are a few examples of facial implants? _____
_____

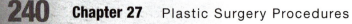

2. What procedures can a facial implant be partnered with? _____

_____

3. Describe a facial implant procedure: _____

_____

_____

_____

_____

_____

BREAST IMPLANTS (AUGMENTATION MAMMAPLASTY)

Answer the following questions.

1. What is the technical name for breast implants? _____

2. Why do women get breast implants? _____

_____

_____

3. Describe a breast implant surgery: _____

_____

_____

4. Why would a woman need to postpone breast implant surgery? _____

_____

5. What happens before the procedure? _____

_____

_____

_____

_____

6. What type of breast cancer screening might happen prior to a procedure?

_____

BREAST-LIFT (MASTOPEXY)

Answer the following questions.

1. Who is a good candidate for a breast-lift? _____

_____

_____

_____

_____

2. A breast-lift involves what types of incisions? _____

_____

3. What are the pre-procedure considerations of this surgery? _____

_____

_____

_____

BREAST REDUCTION (REDUCTION MAMMAPLASTY)

Answer the following questions.

1. Who are good candidates for breast reduction? _____

_____

2. What medical symptoms might a woman have from having pendulous breasts?

a. _____

b. _____

c. _____

d. _____

e. _____

f. _____

g. _____

h. _____

i. _____

j. _____

3. How is the surgery different than mastopexy? _____

_____

4. What type of pre-procedure considerations should there be? _____

_____

_____

_____

BREAST RECONSTRUCTION

Answer the following questions.

1. Who is a good candidate for breast reconstruction? _____
_____

2. Why should clients who smoke quit prior to the procedure? _____
_____

3. Where is an implant inserted? _____

4. How does a surgeon perform a skin expansion plus breast implant procedure?
_____
_____
_____
_____
_____

5. Describe a distant or flap reconstruction: _____
_____
_____
_____
_____

6. Describe a musculocutaneous flap: _____
_____
_____
_____
_____

7. Describe the free flap: _____
_____
_____
_____
_____

8. Explain postoperative activity after a breast implant procedure: _____
_____
_____
_____
_____

9. What risks are involved in breast reconstruction? _____
_____

TUMMY TUCK (ABDOMINOPLASTY)

Answer the following questions.

1. What is the technical name for a tummy tuck? _____

2. What benefits does a tummy tuck offer? _____

_____

3. What is another surgery that would complement a tummy tuck? _____

4. What are the pre-procedure considerations? _____

_____

_____

_____

5. Describe a mini-abdominoplasty: _____

_____

_____

_____

_____

_____

6. Describe a full abdominoplasty: _____

_____

_____

_____

_____

_____

_____

_____

LIPOSUCTION (SUCTION-ASSISTED LIPOPLASTY)

Answer the following questions.

1. What are the other names for liposuction? _____

_____

2. In what areas would a patient receive liposuction? _____

_____

3. What is cellulite? _____

_____

_____

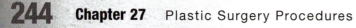

4. What is the name of the tool used to perform liposuction? _____

5. What are the pre-procedure considerations? _____
_____

6. What are advantages of laser-assisted liposuction? _____
_____

7. What is mesotherapy used for? _____
_____

PUTTING IT ALL TOGETHER

Draw a line from the term to its definition.

rhinoplasty   alters the shape of the breast

circumareolar   the top profile of the nose

bariatric surgery   stretch marks

liposuction   refers to a nose job

mammaplasty   refers to a tummy tuck

rhytidectomy   refers to eyelid surgery

blepharoplasty   refers to a face-lift

dorsum   refers to a breast-lift

abdominoplasty   refers to the circumference of the areola

striae distensae   removing stubborn areas of fat

mastopexy   gastric bypass surgery

Date: _____

Rating: _____

PRE-MEDICAL OR LASER INTERVENTION PROCEDURES

Find the following terms in the word search puzzle below.

ablative   Famir   facial
Aquaphor   liposuction   rosacea
Cipro   lymphatic

```
A  C  B  I  N  D  J  P  T  J  X  Y  Q  O  N  L  D  P  B  A
B  B  P  R  D  D  S  O  A  L  H  Z  W  D  X  I  K  I  S  J
L  Z  S  P  Q  P  Y  X  J  Q  Q  R  Q  I  W  X  E  K  Q  M
A  D  F  V  H  P  M  C  L  Y  M  P  H  A  T  I  C  J  M  P
T  P  L  V  A  D  C  I  R  Q  J  S  C  V  O  X  H  E  Q  L
I  G  G  K  H  H  G  G  E  I  Q  B  P  Y  R  T  G  J  N  L
V  C  L  F  L  E  S  E  T  P  M  P  Y  Q  V  T  H  T  T  O
E  V  V  I  I  E  S  E  B  B  N  A  F  Z  A  Z  Q  F  P  N
R  W  W  Q  P  J  M  H  G  H  H  Y  F  L  K  Q  R  M  G  C
Q  P  K  X  X  O  N  K  P  X  P  W  H  H  I  E  Z  H  J  A
W  G  N  Z  H  O  S  I  I  P  Z  O  A  R  U  E  I  W  M  E
C  U  K  R  G  F  O  U  H  K  N  U  O  P  F  N  U  U  T  C
Z  J  A  V  I  A  T  W  C  R  T  H  W  X  V  F  F  C  Z  A
B  R  U  V  O  C  J  W  U  T  P  X  W  T  X  F  H  D  K  S
J  Q  L  R  W  I  Y  Y  O  A  I  S  L  K  B  K  Q  O  P  O
I  F  P  V  N  A  Z  O  U  W  G  O  V  A  C  K  Y  T  C  R
B  I  T  Q  Z  L  E  Q  N  Q  M  K  N  Z  C  V  J  N  H  C
C  L  T  Z  P  C  A  S  H  Z  W  H  B  I  K  K  S  L  R  T
```

1. How will the skin react to the procedure if the skin is in good condition prior to the procedure? _____

_____

2. Name the various facial plastic surgeries:

_____

3. What are various types of ablative laser procedures? _____

_____

4. How does the skin react to laser procedures? _____

_____

5. What should be happening at least two weeks prior to a laser treatment? _____

_____

6. What determines the treatment plan? _____

_____

7. List clinic treatments that an esthetician can perform:

   a. _____

   b. _____

   c. _____

   d. _____

   e. _____

   f. _____

   g. _____

8. Use the words in the word bank to complete the paragraph below.

AHA	progressively
BHA	retinoic acid
Exfoliating	salicylic acid
Jessner's	skin lightening
	traumatizing

Peels include _____, _____, retinoic acid, _____, or _____; select a peel starting with the lowest concentration and gradually increase in strength as the client tolerates. These treatments help to stimulate the home-care program by _____ the upper layers of the epidermis and serve as an additional _____ measure. It is important to make sure the client stops using home-care AHAs, _____, or scrubs one to two days before and three to five days after a peel, depending on its strength. Follow manufacturer's guidelines and avoid being too aggressive, which may result in _____ the skin. This is your time to use your experience, education, and critical-thinking skills to improve the client's skin; with your help, his or her skin can become _____ better in tone and texture, and the client will not have to deal with possible side effects or complications of any procedure.

9. Describe microdermabrasion. _____
_____
_____
_____

10. What should a client stop using prior to a microdermabrasion treatment?
_____
_____

11. Who should not receive a microdermabrasion treatment? _____
_____
_____

ENZYMES

Answer the following questions.

1. What type of enzymes are there?

   a. _____

   b. _____

   c. _____

   d. _____

2. Where does the enzyme papain come from? _____

3. What benefits do enzymes offer? _____
_____

4. Describe ultrasonic technology: _____
_____

5. How does the ultrasonic treatment differ from microdermabrasion? _____
_____

6. What is the exfoliation stage called? _____

7. What is the hydrating stage called? _____

8. During which stage would beneficial serums penetrate? _____

9. Describe microcurrent facial toning: _____
_____
_____

10. How often would a client need to receive microcurrent facial toning treatments?
_____

11. Describe lymph drainage. _____
_____

12. What are the benefits of lymph drainage? _____
_____

13. When is lymph drainage commonly performed? _____
_____

PRE-SURGICAL HOME CARE

Answer the following questions.

1. Prior to a procedure, what should the client be doing at home? _____
_____

2. What would a pre-laser home-care kit focus on? _____

3. List the items in a pre-laser home-care kit:

a. _____

b. _____

c. _____

d. _____

e. _____
_____

4. What are the home-care directions for the morning?

a. _____

b. _____

c. _____

d. _____

5. What are the home-care directions for the evening?

a. _____

b. _____

c. _____

d. _____

6. Use the words in the word bank to complete the paragraph below.

classification	optimum
exfoliate	protect
laser resurfacing	treatment plans

As with _____ or other cosmetic procedures, the client will tolerate the post-surgical phase much better if his or her skin is in _____ condition. If the client is having a combination of procedures, you need to combine both _____. Depending on skin type and _____, clients need to use, at a minimum, products designed to _____, hydrate, condition, and _____.

7. Name the key ingredients in the following products:

a. Cleansers: _____

b. Exfoliators: _____

c. Hydrators/moisturizers: _____

_____

d. Eye creams: _____

e. Sunscreen: _____

AFTER CO$_2$/ERBIUM ND: YAG LASER RESURFACING

1. Explain what happens during the first five days after the procedure: _____

_____

_____

_____

_____

2. Explain what happens during days 5 to 10 after the procedure: _____

_____

_____

_____

_____

_____

_____

_____

3. Days 10 to 30 after the procedure: _____

_____

_____

4. One month post-laser: _____

_____

_____

_____

AFTER A RHYTIDECTOMY OR FACE-LIFT

1. Explain what happens during the first week after surgery: _____

_____

_____

_____

_____

_____

2. Days 8 to 15 after surgery: _____

_____

_____

_____

_____

_____

_____

_____

3. Two weeks after surgery: _____

_____

_____

_____

_____

_____

_____

_____

4. Three weeks or more after surgery: _____

_____

_____

_____

_____

_____

BLEPHAROPLASTY

1. Explain what happens during days 1 to 7 after surgery: _____

_____

_____

_____

_____

_____

_____

_____

_____

_____

_____

2. Days 7 to 12 after surgery: _____

_____

_____

_____

_____

3. Two to three weeks after surgery: _____

_____

_____

_____

4. Two to six months after surgery: _____

_____

_____

JOWL/NECK/CHIN LIPOSUCTION

1. Explain what happens one to three days after surgery: _____

_____

_____

_____

_____

2. Day 4 to four weeks after surgery: _____

_____

_____

_____

_____

_____

_____

_____

3. Four weeks or more after surgery: _____

_____

_____

_____

WHEN TO REFER BACK TO A PHYSICIAN

Answer the following questions.

1. When would a consultation with a physician be needed? _____

_____

_____

_____

_____

2. Draw a line matching the following terms to their definitions.

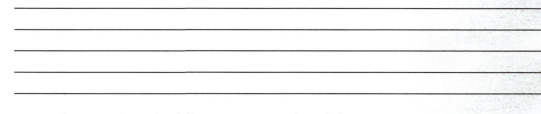

allergic reaction	Skin lightener
Famvir	Eyelid surgery
collagen shrinkage	Removal of fatty deposits
contact dermatitis	Antiviral medication
blepharoplasty	Formation of new epidermis
hydroquinone	Using a CO_2 or Erbium laser
laser resurfacing	A localized skin reaction caused from contact with a substance
liposuction	An abnormal reaction and hypersensitivity
reepithelization	Thermal heating can break down the collagen

Date: _____

Rating: _____

CALCULATING BUSINESS RISK

Answer the following questions.

1. What does *risk* refer to? _____

_____

2. What is a business plan? _____

_____

_____

THE BUSINESS PLAN

1. Fill in the missing components in this business plan.

I. Executive Summary

    a. _____

    b. _____

    _____

    c. _____

II. Marketing Strategy

    a. _____

    b. _____

    c. _____

    d. _____

    e. _____

    _____

III. Strategic Design and Development

    a. _____

b. _____

c. _____

d. _____

e. _____

f. _____

IV. Operations

a. _____
_____

b. _____

c. _____

d. _____

e. _____

f. _____

g. _____

h. _____
_____
_____

V. Financial Information

a. _____

b. _____

c. _____

d. _____

e. _____
_____

f. _____
_____

g. _____

h. _____

2. What should an executive summary state? _____

_____

3. What should the marketing plan section state? _____

_____

_____

_____

4. What should the strategic design and development plan state? _____

_____

_____

_____

_____

5. What should the operations plan state? _____

_____

_____

_____

_____

6. What should the financial plan state? _____

_____

_____

7. What should the conclusion section state? _____

_____

_____

_____

FINANCIAL PLANNING

Answer the following questions.

1. What does _capital_ mean? _____

_____

2. What is a venture capitalist? _____

_____

3. What is a promissory note? _____

_____

4. What is the SBA and what does it do? _____

_____

5. What resources does the SBA offer? _____

_____

FINANCIAL TOOLS

Answer the following questions.

1. What are the financial reports designed to help you manage finances with your accountant?

_____

2. What is a balance sheet? _____

_____

3. What are assets? _____

4. What are liabilities? _____

_____

_____

5. What is owner's equity? _____

_____

_____

6. What is an income statement? _____

_____

_____

_____

7. How do you total up the net profit? _____

_____

8. What is the cash flow statement? _____

_____

9. What is a break-even analysis? _____

_____

PROTECTING BUSINESS ASSETS

Answer the following questions.

1. What is risk management? _____

2. What type of insurance should you have?

a. _____

b. _____

c. _____

d. _____

e. _____

f. _____

g. _____

EMPLOYEE COMPENSATION

Answer the following questions.

1. What are the different ways to compensate employees?

a. _____

b. _____

c. _____

2. How should you report tips to the IRS? _____

3. What is an independent contractor? _____

_____

4. What are the three general categories that determine independent contractor status?

a. _____

b. _____

c. _____

5. Where can you find more information on these three categories? _____

_____

_____

6. If you are an independent contractor, who pays your taxes? _____

UNDERSTANDING THE IRS

Answer the following questions.

1. What is a Social Security Number? _____

2. What is an Employer Identification Number? _____

_____

3. What is an Individual Tax Identification Number? _____

_____

_____

4. What is the W-4 form for? _____

_____

5. What is the W-2 form for? _____

_____

_____

6. What is the I-9 form for? _____

_____

7. What tax form does an independent contractor receive? _____

8. By what date do taxes need to be paid? _____

9. What are the names of the payroll tax deductions? _____

_____

10. What other very important tax are employers responsible for paying?

_____

11. What is a self-employment tax? _____

_____

_____

_____

12. If you make estimated payments four times a year, what form should you use?

_____

13. Define resale tax: _____

_____

14. What is the deferred income tax? _____

_____

_____

15. Explain tax penalties: _____

_____

_____

_____

PUTTING IT ALL TOGETHER

Answer the following questions.

1. It is a type of note that defines the terms of a loan. _____

2. It is the chance of incurring some type of harm. _____

3. It is a statement that indicates how much money is flowing in and out of a business on a regular basis. _____

4. It provides protection against business casualties. _____

5. It is the type of profit that is the total amount of money a business takes in from the sale of products and services. _____

6. If you have your own business, you are an _____ contractor.

7. It is the amount of money invested in a business. _____

8. They are due by April 15th. _____

9. It is a type of analysis that states the point at which all costs are covered and your business begins to earn a profit. _____

10. It is what provides a financial overview of a business at a given point in time in terms of its assets and liabilities. _____

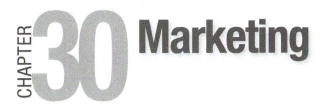

30 **Marketing**

Date: _____

Rating: _____

THE DEFINITION OF MARKETING

Answer the following questions.

1. Explain the basic principles of marketing: _____
_____

2. What happens during the process of marketing? _____
_____

3. What are the Four Ps in Marketing? _____

4. What does *Product* mean? _____
_____
_____
_____

5. What does the business of skin care sell? _____
_____

6. Use the words in the word bank to complete the paragraph below.

brand recognition	medical aesthetic facilities
good public relations	positive
image	product

Image is another significant factor that helps business owners to establish what is referred to as _____. Today's skin care businesses may be housed in any number of facilities, including beauty salons, separate skin care salons, spa-and-salon combinations, or _____. Before you can develop a solid marketing plan, you must decide on the main focus of your business and establish a brand name that embodies the _____ you wish to project. There are other aspects of branding that you should not overlook, such as a _____ program, which will help you to develop a _____ public image. This is all part of developing your "_____."

7. What is one thing that you should consider when it comes to pricing? _____
_____
_____

8. What should your pricing strategy be based on? _____
_____

9. What is a promotion? _____
_____

10. What forms of communication are involved in promotion?

   a. _____

   b. _____

   c. _____

   d. _____

   e. _____

   f. _____

11. To what does *Place* refer? _____
_____
_____
_____
_____
_____

CUSTOMER VALUE

Answer the following questions.

1. What is a consumer? _____

2. What is a seller? _____
_____

3. What are demographics? _____
_____
_____
_____

4. Where is one place you can find demographic information? _____
_____

5. Gathering demographic information is an important part of the marketing process. What are the demographics around your school or salon? _____

_____

Ages: _____

Sex: _____

Income: _____

Education level: _____

Spending habits: _____

6. Given the demographics in your area, what skin care products could you sell easily to every client? _____

CUSTOMER RELATIONSHIP MANAGEMENT

Answer the following questions.

1. In what do smart business owners invest a great deal of time? _____

_____

_____

2. Create a moisturizing product. It can contain various beneficial ingredients and can be priced at any range. Describe the product below: _____

_____

_____

_____

What are its benefits? _____

What is the price? _____

Ask 10 people if they would buy this product and how much they would spend. Record your results.

Person #1 _____

Person #2 _____

Person #3 _____

Person #4 _____

Person #5 _____

Person #6 _____

Person #7 _____

Person #8 _____

Person #9 _____

Person #10 _____

3. What would a total quality management program include? _____

_____

_____

_____

4. Give an example of good customer service that you have had in the past:

_____

5. What is one tool you can use to help you continually evaluate your skin care methods?

_____

THE PROMOTION MIX

Answer the following questions.

1. What are different ways you can promote your business?

a. _____

b. _____

c. _____

d. _____

e. _____

f. _____

g. _____

h. _____

2. As you establish the best methods for promoting your business, it is often helpful to think in what terms? _____

ADVERTISING

Describe each of the following methods of advertising.

1. Classified ads: _____

_____

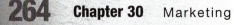

_____

_____

_____

_____

2. Newspaper ads: _____

_____

_____

_____

_____

3. Magazine ads: _____

_____

_____

_____

_____

_____

4. Radio and television ads: _____

_____

_____

_____

_____

5. Direct mail or email ads: _____

_____

_____

_____

_____

_____

_____

6. Rewards programs: _____

_____

_____

7. Activity: Write out an ad for your salon.

_____

_____

_____

_____

PUBLIC RELATIONS

1. List some public relations pieces you can create for a business:

a. _____

b. _____

c. _____

2. What is the benefit of gaining publicity? _____

_____

_____

3. What are some ways you can gain publicity?

a. _____

b. _____

c. _____

d. _____

e. _____

f. _____

4. What type of publicity events can you do for your salon or school in your area?

_____

_____

_____

_____

DIRECT MARKETING

Answer the following questions.

1. Explain direct marketing: _____

_____

_____

2. What are the two important factors in direct marketing? _____

3. Create your own direct mail advertising piece: _____

_____

PERSONAL SELLING

Answer the following questions.

1. What is personal selling? _____

_____

2. What does personal selling require? _____

SALES PROMOTIONS

Answer the following questions.

1. What are the common types of sales promotions? _____

_____

_____

2. What are some creative ways you can bring attention to various salon treatments and products? _____

_____

_____

_____

3. Describe how you would structure a frequent customer/membership program:

_____

THE MARKETING PLAN

Answer the following questions.

1. Your marketing plan should provide a detailed account of all of the marketing methods you will use to achieve your goals. List those marketing methods:

a. _____

b. _____

c. _____

d. _____

e. _____

f. _____

g. _____

2. What are the five primary objectives to consider in marketing skin care?

a. _____

b. _____

c. _____

d. _____

e. _____

3. What should be an ongoing expense in your business? _____

THE BROCHURE, OR MENU OF SERVICES

Answer the following questions.

1. Describe a brochure: _____

_____

_____

_____

_____

2. The brochure should be well-written, organized, and _____.

3. The brochure should be divided into _____.

4. Draw up a brochure of your own.

a. List and describe at least five services you would perform.

1. _____

2. _____

3. _____

4. _____

5. _____

b. Sketch the layout for your brochure on a sheet of letter size paper folded in thirds to create the appearance of a tri-fold brocure.

THE INTERNET

Answer the following questions.

1. What is the Internet? _____

_____

2. Besides having a Web site, what else can you use the Internet for? _____
_____
_____
_____

3. What is the primary goal of any Web site? _____
_____

THE USE OF TECHNOLOGY

Answer the following questions.

1. What can a good salon software program offer? _____
_____
_____

2. Why would you need to track an employee's sales? _____

3. List automatic business builders:

a. _____

b. _____

c. _____

d. _____

e. _____

f. _____

4. There are numerous firms online that will guide the business owner through the process of developing e-marketing materials that allow for "_____" delivery and cost-effectiveness for very nominal fees. All responses can be tracked as can those who "_____". E-newsletters, specials, and birthday wishes are rapidly growing in popularity.

MARKETING RESPONSIBLY

Which government agencies oversee marketing practices, and what do they oversee?

a. _____

b. _____
_____

c. _____
_____

PUTTING IT ALL TOGETHER

Find the chapter's key words below within the word search.

brochure   price

demographic   product

Internet   promotion

marketing   publicity

menu   services

place

```
Y B C D Z E L O O G L S P J V O N O K L
J E Q X D I M E H V A H O Z L C C C Q J
R W T Y R I G T T D G U G A R I Y I P L
J S W U R J G Y C Y M H T O K U M N S U
S P P R O D U C T N P U B L I C I T Y P
T O R O R I L M E N U O X E Q W U E S P
D E M O G R A P H I C F X R W P V R P R
L P Z Q M X X N T N W R Y V M L W N V S
E R G E Q O L E N F S P K W A A R E H S
W G T X N X T N T N J Z E R C Z T N F
U N Z Z D A W I U A R C R V K E H Q T M
F S Z K M L R I O W G U L Z E B R N K X
L A M P B L A A U N H L S Q T D F K C K
N Q M R H I C L B C R N L S I L O O X Z
L P Y Y R V U V O E F U O B N E E H E Z
S Q R V W O K R F C K L F F G C S C O M
V Z C J D U B N W D R O R M L O I N Q L
I M I E R X T S W X N K U Z K R K H O H
Z J Z F W J B R D A P Q F M P U G K C P
Z Y W D X B B S E R V I C E S M Z M L I
```

NOTES

NOTES

NOTES

NOTES

NOTES

NOTES

NOTES

NOTES

NOTES

NOTES